BASIC PROBLEMS IN BURNS

BASIC PROBLEMS IN BURNS

Proceedings of the Symposium for Treatment of Burns held in Prague, Sept. 13—15, 1973.

EDITORS

R. VRABEC, Z. KONÍČKOVÁ,
J. MOSEROVÁ

1975

SPRINGER-VERLAG BERLIN HEIDELBERG NEW YORK

AVICENUM — CZECHOSLOVAK MEDICAL PRESS PRAGUE

Publishers:

AVICENUM, CZECHOSLOVAK MEDICAL PRESS, PRAGUE
SPRINGER VERLAG BERLIN HEIDELBERG NEW YORK

PRINTED IN CZECHOSLOVAKIA BY POLYGRAFIA, PRAGUE

ISBN 3-540-07112-1 SPRINGER-VERLAG BERLIN HEIDELBERG NEW YORK
ISBN 0-387-07112-1 SPRINGER-VERLAG NEW YORK HEIDELBERG BERLIN

PREFACE

This publication comprises the reports presented at the Sýmposium on the Treatment of Burns, held in Prague on September 13–15, 1973 by the Czech Society of Plastic Surgeons under the auspices of the ISBI on the occasion of the 20th anniversary of the foundation of the Prague Burns Unit.

The program of the symposium was confined to four topics which under the present state of burn treatment represent the basic range of clinical problems. They are: surgery of the burn wound, anaesthesiology and resuscitation, septicaemia and complications of the burn illness.

Most of the reports presented at the Symposium are printed in this book in full, as they were submitted by the authors. Only in some cases were the editors obliged to make minor formal adjustments in the interest of the earliest possible publication of the book.

We hope that, after careful study, this publication will arouse the interest of further specialists in such an intricate field as is the treatment of burns and that it will stimulate all those concerned to further work.

We should like to thank all those who facilitated the publication of this book by their participation in the Symposium and by their co-operation.

The Editors

Welcoming Address of the President of the Symposium

On behalf of the organizing committee I would like to welcome all participants in this symposium.

The symposium was organized on the occasion of the 20th anniversary of the foundation of the Prague Burns Unit. Full credit for the establishment of this unit has to be given to Prof. F. Burian (1881–1965), one of the pioneers of plastic surgery and founder of the first plastic surgery department in Czechoslovakia. At this moment all of us pay tribute to him with gratitude and respect.

Through Burian's influence, the treatment of burns was after World War II transferred in this country as well as in most parts of the European continent from the departments of dermatology into the hands of surgeons.

Burian very soon saw the complexity of the problem of treating extensively burned patients and he fully realized that this problem cannot be solved by plastic surgeons alone. A complex problem requires a complex approach by a whole team of specialists from various clinical and theoretical fields and a team of highly trained, devoted nurses. So, in 1953, through Burian's efforts, the Prague Burns Unit was established.

We have been now accumulating experience in the treatment of burns for as long as twenty years. We had many successes and, naturally, also many failures, but we were learning.

We are happy to be able to share our experience with all the participants in this symposium and to have an opportunity to learn more from our guests.

Permit us, once more, to extend to you our sincere welcome. We hope that you will enjoy your stay in Prague.

Professor Helena Pešková, M.D., D.Sc.

CONTENTS

SURGERY OF THE BURN WOUND

THE TACTICS OF NECRECTOMY AND CRAFTING AT THE PRAGUE BURNS CENTRE

R. VRABEC

Department of Plastic Surgery, Charles University, Prague, Czechoslovakia

We selected surgery of the burn wound intentionally as the first theme of our Symposium. The starting point of all pathophysiologic changes in organism is in the burn wound and the plastic surgeons must chiefly endeavour, therefore, to remove the dead tissue as early as possible and to change the open wound in closed one. Many problems are connected with the adherence to this basic principle of surgery and further development of knowledge on wound healing is aiding their solution. There have been considerable changes in the tactics of necrectomy and grafting during the twenty years of existence of this Institute. Modern findings are being introduced into practice, however, general application is rather influenced by the technical equipment available and by the possibilities of the workplace.

Necrectomy

Just as the trend proceeds in the world, with us too, necrectomy is shifting nearer to the accident and radical surgery is extending. We shall hear more today about the methods of early surgical necrectomy and their securing. We do not yet dare ourselves to apply it currently in case of extensive injuries. We are seeking to confront the question of depth of the excision with histologic studies.

We carry out early necrectomy:

1. in case of demarcated contact burns,
2. in case of electric injuries,
3. in case of injuries of hands in hot rollers,
4. in case of extensive injuries in older patients, where radical surgery alone may prevent lethal complications.

Extensive primary excisions require at least two teams of surgeons and the hazards of general anaesthesia are considerable. We conclude necrectomy usually after the second week after the accident. We seek to decrease the possibility of infection to a minimum by applying intensive local therapy.

We try at some indications chemical necrectomy using collagenase. It is often rather difficult to decide upon sulphamylon therapy thus postponing necrectomy. It is not possible under any circumstances to insist dogmatically upon certain procedures; a clinically so variable burns accident must be considered individually.

Grafting

With the development of the grafting instruments this operation also underwent considerable changes. It is not possible today anymore to graft extensive areas by means of Humby's knife and only thin grafts in sheets are the covers of high quality. They can be acquired by means of electro- or sidermatom. These instruments should be a matter of course not only at burns centres but also at all traumatologic workplaces. They afford a simple, rapid and the donor area least damaging collection with the patient and the donor of the skin.

We use for grafting: 1. autografts,
2. allografts – fresh skin,
– frozen skin,
– lyophilized skin,
3. xenografts,
4. synthetic skin.

1. The best means of achieving a satisfactory take is autografting of skin in sheets without gaps. If there was a lack of own skin, we have been using, since 1967, mesh-grafts. Mesh-graft has several advantages due to which it is invaluable. It takes even on an infected wound. The meshes epithelialise rapidly. The grafting period is reduced and the rehabilitation is more rapid. There has been a surprising decrease in the incidence of contractures and the functional results have improved. These grafts are able to conform to unusual contours. The resulting scar is unobtrusive.

2. We cannot imagine any more today extensive burns without allografts. As we have not been able to acquire skins of dead bodies at larger amounts, we do not yet carry out tissue typing. We obtain skin from live donor volunteers and we cover with them the entire granulation area. We do not allow them to take, remove them on the fifth day at the latest, and replace the new ones until autografting is carried out. If they are left for longer, they are difficult to pull away and there is greater bleeding. Thus the skin of up to 15 live donors is required for an extensively burned patient. The collected skin is stored in an ice box at +4 degrees of centigrade. It keeps alive for three weeks.

Lyophilized skin, amnion and chorion are worse biologic dressing. We do not use skin any more at all, we rather use amnion and chorion for covering the donor areas.

3. The large consumption of allografts induced us to use xenografts. We remove the skin of pigs and store it after bacteriologic control, in ice boxes for up to ten days. We are in a position to confirm all the known good experience. In general the indication is identical with allografts. The advantages of both are:

1. they clean up granulating areas,
2. they protect open wounds from water and protein losses,
3. they decrease pain,
4. they decrease bacterial counts,
5. they increase mobility of the patient,
6. they enhance the growth of epithelium.

We observed general reaction after repeated application of pig skin, only exceptionally.

We had even several times the opportunity to test synthetic skin cover, we do not trust its wider application and shall always give preference to biologic cover.

All this experience is well known to our co-workers treating burned patients. Studies of the phenomena in the recipient site and of the possibilities to influence the process of taking, should make the future grafts more successful. There will be also higher demands upon the final look of the graft, the cover will have to be of sufficiently good quality to enable the burned patient to find his place in normal life.

R. V., Dept. of Plastic Surgery,
Legerova 63,
120 00 Praha 2, Czechoslovakia

EXCISION OF ACUTE BURNS WITH IMMEDIATE MESHED AUTOGRAFTING

B. G. MACMILLAN, E. J. LAW and J. P. FIDLER

Shriners Burns Institute, Cincinnati Unit, Cincinnati, Ohio, U.S.A.

Introduction

Multiple attempts to convert large areas of full thickness burns into clean closed wounds by primary excision and immediate autografting in past years have been unsuccessful. The mortality rate of these patients treated by excisional therapy closely approximated that of patients treated by conventional techniques. This was largely because the clean excised wounds could not be closed per primum as a result of local burn wound sepsis. Subsequently, the local sepsis developed into invasive burn wound sepsis, and the same incidence of septic complications was noted as was seen in the conventionally treated groups. During the past ten years, in addition to many technical advances in skin grafting, improved local and systemic supportive measures have evolved and necessitated a reappraisal of excision as a therapeutic measure for treating major burns. These improvements in patient care include the ability to expand skin and close wounds per primum with minimum amounts of autogenous skin, development of specific anti-staphylococcal, gram negative and antifungal local and systemic antibacterial agents, the ability to reinforce the patient's immune response to infection by the use of active and passive immunological techniques, the availability of fresh frozen component blood therapy, improved methods of nutritional support by the oral route, the availability of synthetic skin substitutes for use when allografts and xenografts are not available, tissue typing techniques to prolong the usefulness of allografts, and the ability to selectively differentiate between viable and nonviable tissue by the Janzekovic technique.

Material and Methods

This re-evaluation was started in 1964 and consists of a group of children ranging in age from 1 to 14 years, with a mean age of 7 years. The extent of total body burn ranged from 4 to 90 percent. Twenty-two of the patients had burns of up to 29 percent of their total body surface, 21 had burns of up to 59 percent, and 15 had burns in excess of 60 percent of the total body surface. The surgical techniques for removing areas of full thickness burn consisted of sharp dissection as described by MacMillan, avulsion as described by Herman, tangential excision as described by Janzekovic, and the laser technique as described by Fidler.

Sharp dissection was used to excise the burn wounds of 15 patients, avulsion for 12 patients, tangential excision for 17 patients, and the laser technique for 14 patients. Electro-surgical excision of portions of the burn eschar in the laser group was used in 3 patients.

In the group of 15 patients treated by sharp dissection, the mean area of total body burn was 40 percent and the mean area of full thickness injury was 28 percent. The mean day of excision was the 12th postburn day. A mean of 20 percent of the total body surface was excised at the first excisional procedure. Two patients had 2 excisional procedures and 1 patient had 3, at which times a mean of 7 and 5 percent, respectively, were removed. The mean blood loss during the first excisional procedure was 330 ccs, during the second procedure, 340 ccs, and during the third, 100 ccs. These blood losses represent 14, 15 and 4 percent of the total blood volume, respectively. Initial coverage of the excised wounds was accomplished with autogenous tissue in 6 patients, with allografts in 1 patient, and with xenografts in 5. A group of 6 patients had their wounds covered initially with gentamicin occlusive dressings. A mean of 3 autogenous procedures were required to accomplish this wound coverage. During this interval, a mean of 1 application of allografts and 3 applications of xenografts were used in conjunction with autogenous coverage. The mean postburn day of total coverage was the 38th, and the mean day of discharge was the 77th postburn day. In this group of 15 patients, 6 were able to maintain their weight by hyperalimentation during the grafting period. Nine patients had a mean weight loss of 12 percent of their total body weight when wound coverage was completed.

In the group of 12 patients treated by the avulsion technique, the mean total body burn was 61 percent, and the mean area of full thickness injury was 54 percent. The mean postburn day of the first excisional procedure was the 12th, at which time a mean of 20 percent of the total body surface was excised. Seven patients underwent a second excisional procedure at which time a mean of 10 percent of the total body surface was excised approximately one week following the first procedure. Two patients had a third excisional procedure, and two a fourth, again at weekly intervals, involving a mean excision of 5 per cent at each operation. Initial coverage was accomplished with autogenous tissue in 8 patients, none were covered with allografts and 3 with xenografts, while occlusive dressings were used to close the wounds in 1 patient. A mean of 6 autografting procedures were required to accomplish wound coverage by the 71st mean postburn day. During this period, a mean of 2 allograft and 5 xenograft procedures were used to maintain wound closure. The mean day of discharge occurred in this group on the 104th postburn day. The mean blood loss of 580 ccs occurred during the first procedure, 397 ccs during the second, 325 during the third, and 500 during the 4th. The mean per cents of blood volume lost during the first, second, third and fourth procedures were 24, 17, 13 and 22 per cent, respectively. Two of the 12 patients were able to maintain their weight through the grafting period; however, 10 patients lost a mean of 18 per cent of their total body mass during the grafting period.

In the group of 17 patients treated by the tangential technique, the mean area of total body burn was 46 per cent and the mean area of full thickness burn was 32 per cent. The mean day of the first excisional procedure was the 9th postburn day. A mean of 16 percent of the total body surface was excised at the first excisional procedure. Six patients underwent 2 excisional procedures with a mean area of 9 per cent being excised, 3 patients underwent 3 procedures with a mean excision of 5 per cent, and 2 patients had 4 procedures with a mean excision of 9 per cent. The mean blood loss during the first excisional procedure was 592 ccs, during the second procedure, 387 ccs, 362 ccs during the third procedure, and 500 ccs during the fourth procedure. This represents a mean percent of total blood volume loss occurring during the first, second, third and fourth procedures of 26, 17, 16 and 22 per cent, respectively. The initial coverage of the excised wounds was accomplished with autogenous tissue in 7 patients, with xenografts in 4, and with silver sulfadiazine occlusive dressings in 5 patients, supplemented with a mean of 4 allograft and 3 xenograft procedures. A mean of 3 autografting procedures were required to accomplish wound coverage. The mean postburn day of total coverage was the 32nd, and the mean day of discharge was the 79th postburn day. Five of the 17 patients maintained their body weight with intensive oral nutritional support, and a group of 12 of the 17 lost a mean of 13 per cent of their total body weight by the time of wound closure.

In the group of 14 patients treated by laser excision, the mean area of total body burn was 23 per cent, and the mean area of full thickness injury was 17 per cent. The mean day of excisional therapy was the 7th postburn day. A mean of 11 per cent of the total body surface was excised at the first excisional procedure, and 4 patients underwent a second procedure with the laser scalpel approximately one week later, at which time 5 per cent of their total body surface was removed. The mean blood loss at the first and second procedures was 316 ccs and 62 ccs, respectively. This mean blood loss represents 14 and 3 per cent of the total blood volume. The initial coverage of the excised wounds was accomplished with autogenous tissue in all 14 patients. A mean of 3 autogenous procedures were necessary to accomplish wound coverage, these being complemented with a mean of 1 application of xenografts. The mean postburn day of total coverage was the 22nd day, and the mean day of discharge was the 58th postburn day. Five of the 14 patients maintained their weight with oral hyperalimentation, the mean weight loss in the other 9 patients in the group representing 11 per cent of their total body weight.

Discussion

Septic complications were encountered in 24 per cent of this group of 58 patients. Burn wound sepsis was encountered in 17 per cent, cardiovascular complications in 36 percent, pulmonary complications in 7 per cent, and gastrointestinal complications in 7 per cent of the patients. The organisms most commonly recovered from the proven cases of septicemia were the gram negative *Pseudomonas aeruginosa* and the yeast *Candida albicans*. One of the patients developed burn wound sepsis in the excised area, and 9 in the unexcised area. The most common cardiovascular complication was hypertension, which was documented in 9 patients. Pulmonary edema was noted in 5 patients, while 2 patients sustained cardiac arrests, both of whom were resuscitated without sequelae. Two patients developed pulmonary emboli, one patient required heparin therapy for thrombophlebitis, and one patient developed congestive heart failure. The most common pulmonary complication which was encountered in 7 patients was pneumonia, and 1 patient developed a pneumothorax as a result of a misplaced central venous pressure catheter.

In a group of 4 patients, renal complications were present, consisting of acute tubular necrosis in 2, nephrosis in 1 and renal lithiasis in 1. Four patients developed gastrointestinal complications. Two patients bleeding from Curling's ulcer responded to conservative therapy, 1 patient developed a duodenal ulcer under therapy, and 1 patient developed an esophageal stricture as a result of a feeding esophageal enterostomy tube.

Three deaths occurred in this group, 1 in the group with 30 to 59 per cent total body burns and 2 in the group with burns in excess of 60 per cent of the total body surface. There was 1 death in each of the sharp, avulsion and tangential groups, one of these resulting from pulmonary emboli and 2 from *Candida albicans* septicemia. The per cent of total body burn represented by the deaths was 44, 90 and 87 per cent, respectively, and the postburn day of death was the 36th, the 26th and the 55th day, respectively. The overall mortality rate in this series was 5 per cent.

The success from this re-evaluation of excisional therapy can be attributed to the ability now to accomplish early permanent wound closure, this largely being made possible by the use of expansion meshed grafts from autogenous tissue placed over the areas of excision. In those patients treated by the tangential technique of Janzekovic, allografts were used to cover all areas of excised deep dermal burn, and autogenous tissue to cover areas of full thickness injury. In those patients who developed burn wound sepsis from either gram positive, gram negative or yeast organisms, specific antibiotics were administered intravenously.

This experience substantiates the fact that excisional therapy is indicated for the removal of large areas of full thickness burn so that postburn morbidity and mortality can be decreased.

B. G. M., 202 Goodman St.,
Cincinnati, Ohio 45219, U.S.A.

EARLY EXCISION OF THIRD-DEGREE BURNED SKIN AREAS UNDER BIOPTICAL CONTROL

A. BERGER, G. MEISSL and H. MILLESI

Department for Plastic and Reconstructive Surgery, First Surgical Clinic, University of Vienna, Austria

Early excision of necrotic tissue is of course the method of choice in third-degree burns. It is, however, often difficult to estimate the degree of damage to the injured tissue before or during surgery. Especially in the first days after a burn it is difficult to distinguish living and necrotic tissue also by normal light microscopic methods. It is also often impossible in the early post-burn period to precisely estimate the depth and extent of deep second-degree burn marks and third-degree burns. It is therefore highly important to have reliable methods for estimating the necrotic and healthy tissue. Some of these are using dye, others isotopes or oxytetracycline, and some thermographic methods. But all these above-mentioned methods have in our opinion certain disadvantages. This point should be discussed later.

Method and material

To find out, within a minimum period of time, the viability of a quite definite layer during an operation, a method is used which is based on the diagnosis of the activity of a definite enzyme. This oxidizing enzyme can be found only in viable cells. Its activity is lost when the cells undergo devitalization.

For our method, we selected the activity and estimation of the enzyme diphosphopyridine nucleotide diaphorases (DPND-D). This ferment can be found in living cells. If diphosphopyridine nucleotide in reduced state in the presence of nitrotetrazolium blue chloride reacts with DPND, there occurs a bluish staining of the tissue (Fig. 1). No blue staining can be detected if the cells of the probe are not any more alive. Under normal condition, no enzyme activity can be consequently seen in the stratum corneum of the epidermis. In this layer of the dermis, no living cells are normally present. By placing a biopsy into a test solution for five to ten minutes one gets precise information on the places in which the DPND activity of the enzyme has vanished and where a necrosis has therefore to be taken into account. This reaction — the blue colour — can be seen without using a magnifying glass or a microscope (Fig. 2).

The test solution consists of 1.0 ml reduced diphosphopyridine nucleotide at a concentration of 2.5 mg/ml and 2.5 ml nitrotetrazolium blue chloride at a concentration of

2.0 mg/ml and 1.0 ml phosphate buffer solution at a concentration of 2.0 mg/ml and 0.5 ml lactated Ringer solution.

The ingredients of this test solution are available in every histological laboratory. This solution has to be prepared the same day it will be used. For use during surgery, small

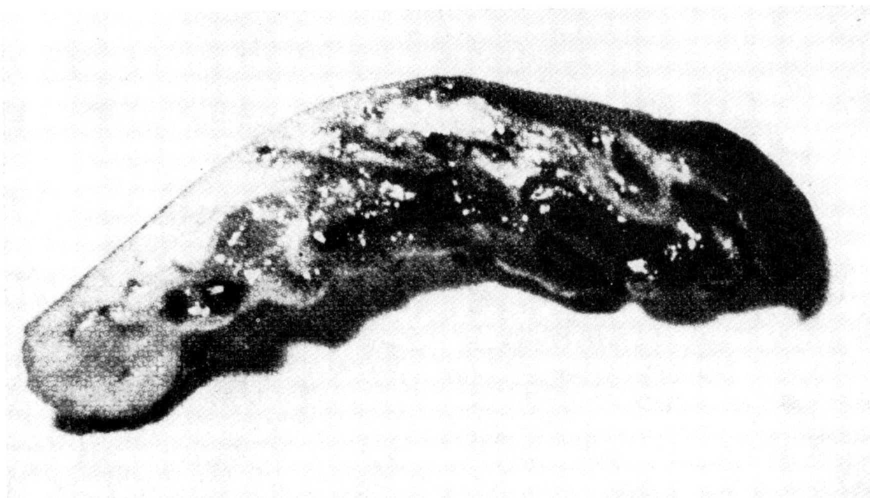

Fig. 1. DPND-stained biopsy of skin and fatty tissue showing the border between necrosis and living tissue.

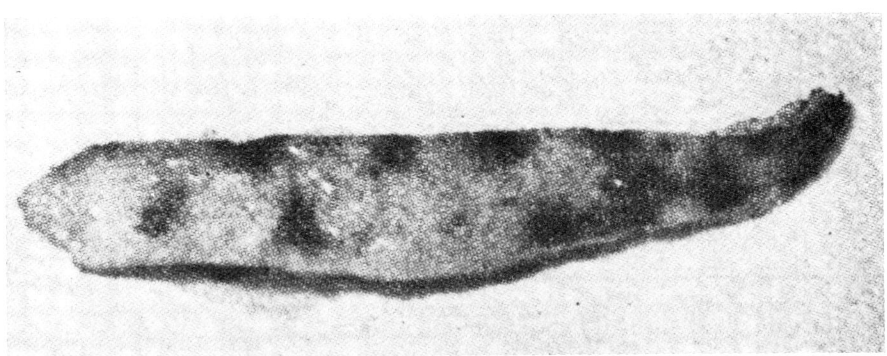

Fig. 2. DPND-stained biopsy from fatty tissue and fascia demonstrating only points of activity. Also this biopsy has to be treated like a necrosis.

portions of the solution are given into small bowls. These small containers are sterilized. To make an estimation of necrotic tissue, one has only to take a biopsy of the questionable part of the tissue and to place it in the test solution. Five to ten minutes later it is possible to define the border between the necrosis and living tissues. For later histological preparation the biopsy in a 5.0 formaline solution can be taken.

If the biopsy is stained blue, the cells are alive, if the probe shows only some sprinkles of bluish colour or no colouring, necrotic tissue is present and has therefore to be excised. This method makes it especially easy to decide whether fatty tissue, fascia, tendons or nerves are alive. This applies especially to tissues in the deeper layers of the injured part after a thermal trauma.

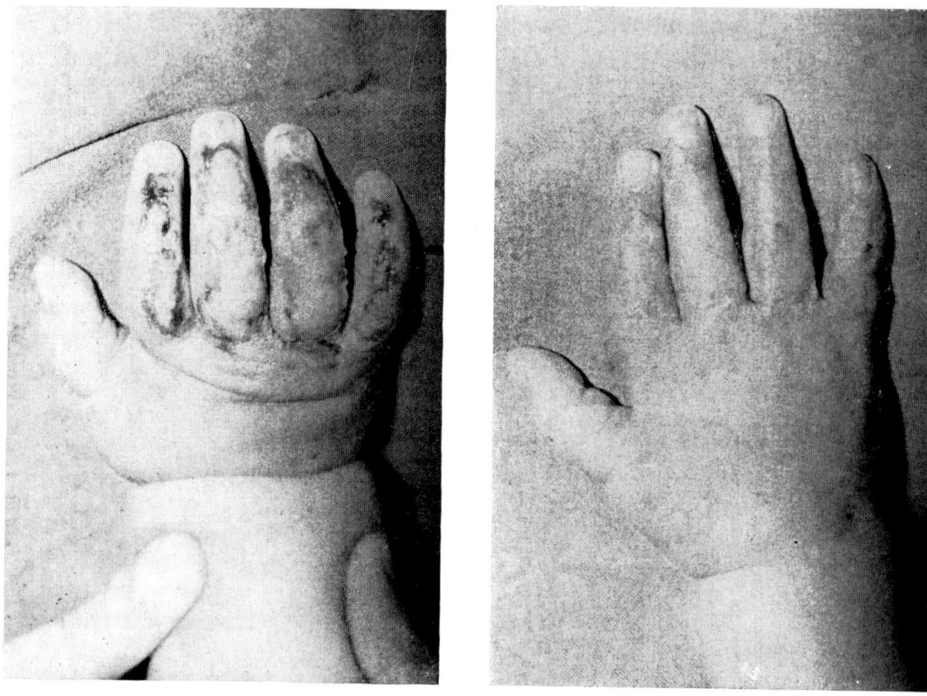

Fig. 3. A — 2-year-old boy with third-degree burn on the dorsum of the hand. Using DPND the early excision was performed and the tendons could be preserved. B — Picture to the right shows the hand one month after the injury.

This method has been used in our department since 1967 and since that time more reliable excisions and therefore early surgery in cases of burns have been performed. Especially on the hands it is possible to operate as early as possible and to excise as much tissue as necessary. Better functional results can therefore be obtained (Fig. 3). This picture demonstrates one of these cases.

Discussion

If one is convinced that early excision of necrotic tissue, especially in third-degree burns, is the method of choice, one must also know the problems involved in estimating the extent of the necrosis and especially its depth. Intravenous injection of a dye makes it possible to distinguish between partial and full thickness skin loss following burns. The dye produces a vital staining in full vascularised tissue. Regions without blood-supply remain unstained, so that the line of demarcation can be seen on the surface between necrosis and partial skin damage. The main drawback of this method of vital staining is however, that it does not show the extent of the depth of the necrosis. Knowledge of this is, however, most important in an early excision.

The methods using isotopes have the same disadvantages. As regards the use of oxytetracycline, we found in a study that very often the extent of necrosis shown by this method did not agree with the necrosis detected by the histological and DPND method. Therefore the method based on the diagnosis of the activity of a definite enzyme is in our opinion at present the most reliable and easiest to be handled. Especially for early excision on the hands and other important parts of an injured body it is possible to decide in minimum time whether the tissue is necrotic or alive, so that fascia or tendons or nerves can be preserved and better primary treatment is given for the rehabilitation of a burned patient.

References

1. Bennet, J. E. and Dingmann, O. (1957): Evaluation of burn depth by the use of radioactive isotopes. Plast. reconstr. Surg. 20 : 261.
2. Berger, A. und Sponer, D. (1971): Markierungsmethoden bei Verbrennungen zweiten und dritten Grades. Act. Chir. 6 : 285.
3. Cope, O., Langohr, J. L., Moore, F. D. and Webster, R. L. (1947): Expeditious care of full thickness burn wounds by surgical excision and grafting. Ann. Surg. 125 : 1.
4. Dingwall, J. A. (1943): A clinical test for differentiating second from third degree burn. Plast. reconstr. Surg. 118 : 427.
5. Geldmacher, J. und Scranowitz, P. (1969): Die frühzeitige diagnostische Abgrenzung zweit- und drittgradiger Verbrennungen unter besonderer Berücksichtigung der verbrannten Hand. Med. Welt 20 : 3.
6. Lechner, G. und Millesi, H. (1967): Fermentreaktion zur Bestimmung der Tiefe des Gewebsschadens bei Verbrennungen. Act. Chir. 2 : 221.
7. Málek, P., Dobrovský, Zástava, V. and Kolc, J. (1963): The proposed use of tetracycline antibiotics for the evaluation of the degree of burns. Acta Chir. plast. 5 : 48.
8. Millesi, H. (1970): Fermentreaktion und Vitalitätsprüfung. Chir. plast. reconstr. 8 : 43.

A. B., 1st Surgical Clinic,
Alserstr. 4,
1090 Wien, Austria

SURVIVAL OF SEVERELY BURNED PATIENTS WITH INTERMEDIATE DURATION SKIN TRANSPLANTATION AND IMMUNOSUPPRESSION

R. K. J. KOUMANS, P. S. RUSSELL and J. F. BURKE

The Surgical Services, Zuiderziekenhuis, Rotterdam; the Massachusetts General Hospital and Shriners Burns Institute, Harvard Medical School, Boston

Introduction

Despite recent advances in topical burn therapy, experience continues to record that patients with extensive full-thickness skin loss, exceeding 60 per cent or more of body surface, have almost no chance of survival. Death eventually supervenes, not caused by the thermal injury in itself, nor simply as a result of infection, but by an irreversible catabolic state, related to the prolonged insufficiency of a vital organ: the intact integument.

Early removal of dead tissue and closure of the wound — one of the oldest axioms and aims of surgery — will prevent these secondary pathological problems and provide in our view the only means of improving decisively the mortality due to very extensive burns.

However this therapeutic principle — well accepted as it is in treating full thickness burns of limited size — could not be applied in these patients as the extent of skin loss present logistic problems that cannot be solved by contemporary methods of skin replacement. A possible solution to this problem can be found in skin allo-transplantation (4).

Viable skin allografts from random donors are rejected within 12 days and even if chosen by ABO and HL-A genotype matching, rejection will take place in about 15 days in a parent-to-sibling (one haplotype identical) combination (1). Despite the additional immunosuppressive effect resulting from the debility of an extensive burn, skin allograft survival from similarly matched donors on burned recipients, will seldom last more than 20 days (2). This is not long enough for these patients to heal their limited areas of partial thickness burn in order to serve as donor sites for autografts.

By combining tissue typing and immunosuppresion, we have prolonged the survival of skin transplants to permit burned children, with full thickness skin destruction that has proven lethal in the past, to survive.

Case reports

Case 1.

A 2.5 year old girl was admitted 2 days following extensive burns, when her clothes caught fire. She had a 91 per cent body surface area (BSA) burn, 80 per cent third degree and 11 per cent deep second. Nursing care was carried out from the day of admission — as in all patients reported here — in bacteria controlled nursing units (BCNU) based on a laminar down flow principle (3).

The patient and all available family members were typed for ABO and HL-A compatibility and the most suitable donor was selected. Within a week after admission all full thickness burns on her extremities and the anterior surface of her body had been excised and covered with allografts and available autografts. Immunosuppression was carried out using oral azathioprine (6 mg/kg the day before transplantation, 3 mg/kg for 3 days and 1.5–2 mg/kg daily thereafter). The allografts were stepwise replaced by autografts harvested from regenerated split thickness donor sites and healed areas of second degree burns.

At 10 weeks following injury all anterior surfaces and extremities were closed with autograft and at 14 weeks the patient was sufficiently covered with autologous skin to be removed from the BCNU. She was discharged from the hospital 28 weeks after injury.

Case 2.

A 7 year old boy was admitted with 81 per cent BSA burns (72 per cent third degree and 9 per cent deep second) caused by his burning clothes. Nursing care was carried out in the BCNU and a program of total excision of 3rd degree burns, immediate allotransplantation and immunosuppression was undertaken. The patient and all available family members were tissue-typed and the individual with the best match selected as donor. Immunosuppression was carried out along the same lines as in the first patient.

All excised areas — except parts of the left leg, which were covered with available autograft — were grafted with allogeneic skin. This was subsequently replaced in a stepwise fashion as more autografts became available through donor site regeneration and healing of second degree burns. The patient was sufficiently covered with autograft to leave the bacteria controlled environment 14 weeks following injury and was discharged from hospital 24 weeks after admission.

Case 3.

A 7.5 year old boy incurred a 91 per cent BSA burn (74 per cent third degree and 17 per cent deep second). He was treated along the same lines as the other patients. The entire area of full thickness skin loss was excised in 4 operative sessions and except for a primarily autografted area on the right leg, allografts were applied with excellent take. These allografts were replaced stepwise as autografts became available. The patient was sufficiently covered with his own skin to leave the BCNU 14 weeks post burn and was discharged home 10 weeks later.

Discussion

Skin allo-transplantation provides immediate closure of the wound following primary excision of extensive full thickness burns. In order to be effective in improving patient survival, the transplanted skin must remain viable and functioning long enough to allow for its complete stepwise replacement by autograft. In our experience this procedure requires between 30 and 60 days. To provide adequate graft prolongation moderate dosage immunosuppressive therapy is therefore indispensable. The additional threat of infection posed by immunosuppression was reduced by providing continuous aseptic burn care in bacteria controlled nursing units.

In previous experimental work we have shown that antilymphocyte globulin (ALG) is the immunosuppressive drug of choice for skin transplantation in burns, as it provides good graft prolongation while leaving humoral (anti-bacterial) immunity of the host essentially unaffected (4).

At the time the patients reported here were admitted, we could not dispose of sufficient amounts of adequately tested ALG and azathioprine was used instead. Recently we treated a 6 year old patient with 88 percent BSA burns, of which 9 per cent deep second degree, with skin transplantation and immunosuppression with ALG. Though this patient is still in the hospital, she is now completely covered with autografts and has left the BCNU. It was the impression of all concerned that the ALG provided a superior clinical course as compared with the imuran treated patients.

The concept of transplantation used in the treatment of these patients differs from other organ transplantations in that no attempt is made to achieve permanent survival of the grafts. This policy is based on the unique situation that staged replacement with autologous tissue can be accomplished. At the same time full scale immunosuppression in burn patients seems a hazardous procedure and its long term effect at least doubtful, as skin transplants are known for the ease with which they are rejected. We have therefore used the term "intermediate duration transplantation" to further differentiate this concept from that of the short term use of allografts or xenografts of skin as a biological dressing.

Early excision of full thickness burns and wound closure by intermediate duration skin transplatantion using donor selection, immunosuppression and aseptic patient care in a controlled environment have provided a successful approach in the treatment of the severely injured burn patient.

References

1. Amos, D. B., Seigler, H. F., Southworth, J. G., Ward, F. E. (1969): Skin graft rejection between subjects genotyped for HL-A. Transplant. Proc. 1 : 342.
2. Burke, J. F.: Allograft survival as related to HL-A type in physiologically stable burn patients. Unpublished data.
3. Burke, J. F. (1971): Isolation techniques and their effectiveness. In: Contemporary Burn Management. Ed. by H. C. Polk and H. H. Stone. Little, Brown and Co., Boston, 141.
4. Koumans, R. K. J., Burke, J. F. (1969): Skin allografts and immunosuppression in the treatment of massive thermal injury. Surgery 66 : 89.

R. K. J. K., Zuiderziekenhuis,
Rotterdam 24, The Netherlands

EPIGARD — A NEW SYNTHETIC WOUND DRESSING: COMPARATIVE CLINICAL STUDIES WITH PORCINE XENOGRAFT

H. M. BRUCK

Burn Unit, Harlem Hospital Center, New York, New York, U.S.A.

The uses of cutaneous allograft and xenograft as physiologic membranes to cover and protect granulating burn wounds and to prepare them for definitive isografting are well established (1, 6). Difficulties with procurement of cutaneous allograft and xenograft, short shelf life, antigenicity and high cost limit the value of these physiologic dressings. A synthetic membrane that simulates the properties of human skin would answer these shortcomings.

Numerous synthetic membranes tested over the years have been discarded because of subgraft suppuration, stiffness, poor adherence to the wound, and retained fragments. The most notable of the synthetics which showed early promise include Ivalon sponge (2,4), a membrane of polyvinyl alcohol; amino acid films (5); velours of nylon, rayon and Dacron (3) and thermoplastic vinyl polymers. In addition to the problems of suppuration, retained fragments and non-adherence, there was no control over evaporation.

Against this background, the search continued for the synthetic that most closely met the several "ideal properties" of conformity, adherence, bacteriologic control, long shelf life and low cost.

Epigard, the synthetic described in this report, is a microporous film of polyetrafluoroethylene, a teflon drapelike material, laminated to a thin sheet of reticulated polyurethane foam. The foam side of the dressing acts as a scaffold for adhesion to the wound and ingrowth of fibroblasts and capillaries. The microporous outer membrane is a gas permeable barrier to liquids and bacteria. A comparison study was undertaken between Epigard and porcine xenograft in human burn patients. Predominantly full thickness and a few partial thickness burn wounds, treated initially with topical chemotherapy — i.e., silver-sulfadiazine or mafenide acetate, were selected for study. Epigard and porcine xenograft (either the fresh or fresh-frozen preparation) were placed in juxtaposition on granulating wounds following slough or debridement of eschar. In this way, each patient served as his own control. Xenograft and Epigard were changed daily until the quality of the granulations improved, as manifest by adherence of the dressing, decrease in exudate, and bleeding of the granulating surface. At this time, dressings were changed every two to five days until definitely closed with isograft.

The wounds were monitored by clinical assessment of appearance, improvement and isograft take, surface bacteriology using touch plates, and periodically by biopsy. 24 cases were studied in this manner ranging in age from 11 years to 68 years (average 44.8 years), and in burn size from 3 to 68 percent (average 23 percent) total body surface area burn.

Results

In general, Epigard appeared equal to porcine xenograft in wound appearance, frequently superior in wound adherence and equal in percentage of isograft "takes". Of the cases under study, 16 demonstrated a good graft take in wounds prepared with both porcine xenograft and Epigard; graft loss occurred equally in one patient in both test and control site; in 5 cases, wound deterioration associated with sepsis occurred in all wound sites; and in two cases, surgery for definitive wound closure was refused by the patient. Of interest, in an additional 3 cases, excluded from the study, the resident switched to Epigard as sole wound dressing because he thought the wound looked better beneath it.

Bacteriologic data obtained from the wound surface showed no significant difference in wounds beneath either porcine xenograft or Epigard although sterility was rarely accomplished. Wound biopsies demonstrated no retained fragments.

Conclusions

In these preliminary clinical studies, Epigard appears to be an effective dressing for the granulating wound, equal to porcine xenograft as a temporary biologic dressing and a good debriding agent. Epigard conforms to the wound surface and develops a firm adherence to the wound. Quantitative tissue bacteriology is needed to further define the bacteriostatic properties, if any. More extensive clinical trials are needed to assess the role of Epigard over larger burn surfaces.

References

1. Bromberg, B. E., Song, I. C., Mohn, M. P. (1965): The use of pig skin as a temporary biological dressing. Plast. recontr. Surg. 36 : 80.
2. Chardack, W. M., Brueske, D. A., Santomauro, A. P., Fazekas, G. (1962): Experimental studies on synthetic substitutes for skin and their use in the treatment of burns. Ann. Surg. 155 : 127.
3. Spira, M., Fissette, J., Hall, W. et al. (1969): Evaluation of synthetic fabrics as artificial skin grafts to experimental burn wounds. J. biomed. mat. Res. 3 : 213.
4. Taylor, P. H., Moncrief, J. A., Switzer, W. E., Rose, L. R., Pugsley, L. Q. (1963): Ivalon as a cover for excised burn wounds. Arch. Surg. 86 : 250.
5. Walder, A. I., May, P. D., Bingham, C. P. et al. (1969): Evaluation of synthetic films as wound covers. Trans. Amer. Soc. artif. intern. Org. 15 : 29.
6. Zaroff, L. I., Mills, W., Jr., Duckett, J. W., Jr., Switzer, W. E., Moncrief, J. A. (1966): Multiple uses of viable cutaneous homografts in the burned patient. Surgery 59 : 368.

H. M. B., 161 Fort Washington Ave.,
New York, New York 10032, U.S.A.

TEMPORARY SKIN COVER

G. D. WINTER

Department of Biomedical Engineering, Institute of Orthopaedics, University of London, Royal National Orthopaedic Hospital, Stanmore, Middlesex, Great Britain

Biological dressings range from allografts (homografts), cadaveric or otherwise, through xenografts (zoografts) from pigs, dogs and other species, to embryonic membranes, embryo foetus and neonatal skin, films of reconstituted collagen from bovine and other sources and fibrin.

Originally conceived as temporary dressings for full thickness burn injuries their uses have been extended by some to the treatment of partial thickness burns, tangentially ex-excised burns, mesh grafted burns, donor sites, electrical injuries, traumatic injuries and ulcers.

Advantages claimed for biological dressings are that they:

1. restore a water vapour barrier and prevent dehydration of the wound,
2. decrease evaporational heat loss,
3. decrease protein and electrolyte losses in wound exudate,
4. prevent bacterial colonisation of the wound (3); protect wound and patient from sepsis,
5. decrease pain, facilitating physiotherapy,
6. permit less painful dressing changes, which can often be done on the wards,
7. permit painless movement over joints,
8. facilitate debridement of wounds,
9. improve patients' well being,
10. create good granulation tissue bed for autografting of deep wounds,
11. can be used to test for successful subsequent autograft take,
12. decrease healing time of partial thickness burns and donor sites,
13. improve quality of healing, inhibit excessive fibroplasia, decrease contraction.

The disadvantages of using biological materials as dressings are that they:

1. are troublesome and costly to obtain,
2. are non-uniform,
3. are difficult to sterilise and store aseptically,
4. have a short shelf-life,
5. are potentially antigenic,
6. carry a risk of unusual infection or contaminants,

7. may provoke hypersensitivity to one or more complex constituents,
8. can be abused through familiarity and carelessness,
9. may be unsatisfactory aesthetically.

Freeze dried porcine skin and fresh frozen porcine skin dressings are now available commercially.

There is a persistent but unproven assumption in the literature that biological dressings facilitate wound healing by some unknown mechanism, contributing something that synthetic dressings lack (1, 6).

To circumvent the antigenicity problem it is universally recommended that such dressings are removed daily or at the most every three or four days. Initially the frequent changing of dressings helps to cleanse the burn surface and reduce the bacterial count but the main object is to avoid the immune reaction which is otherwise encountered around the fifth day. In apparant contradiction to this it is said (7, 2) that a major requirement of allografts and xenografts is that they should adhere firmly to the wound and the dressings should act as a scaffolding permitting fibroblasts to invade its structure which implies that some of the foreign dermis will be incorporated into the wound, provoking antigenic and foreign-body reactions. Similar objections can be levelled at open cell foams and other synthetic skin substitute designed to permit tissue ingrowth in that it is impossible to remove the dressings completely without leaving dressing material embedded in the tissues.

The first phase of an investigation designed to study biological dressings was to make observations on autografts, fresh allografts and frozen stored allografts and compare these with occlusive dressings on shallow wounds in the skin of young Large White Pigs.

Materials and Methods

Wounds

2.5 cm × 2.5 cm × approx. 0.5 mm deep in the skin on the backs of female, pedigree Large White Pigs (15–20 weeks old).

Autografts

2.5 cm × 2.5 cm × 0.5 mm thick skin immediately placed on recipient site.

Fresh Allografts

2.5 cm × 2.5 cm × 0.5 mm thick skin from one animal immediately placed on recipient site of second animal.

Stored, frozen allografts

"Zenoderm" porcine skin*, bathed in balanced electrolyte solution, frozen, sterilised by electron irradiation and stored at —76 centigrades.

Occlusive dressings

Polythene: 0.005″ thick natural grade polyethylene film, sterilised by U.V. irradiation.

Results

Shallow wound, no dressing

On the shallow wounds exposed to the air a scab had formed by the end of the first day. The scab contained part of the exposed dermal tissue which, being unprotected by

* The author is grateful to Hancock Laboratories Incorporated, 965 North Trustin Street, Orange, California, U.S.A. for a gift of "Zenoderm".

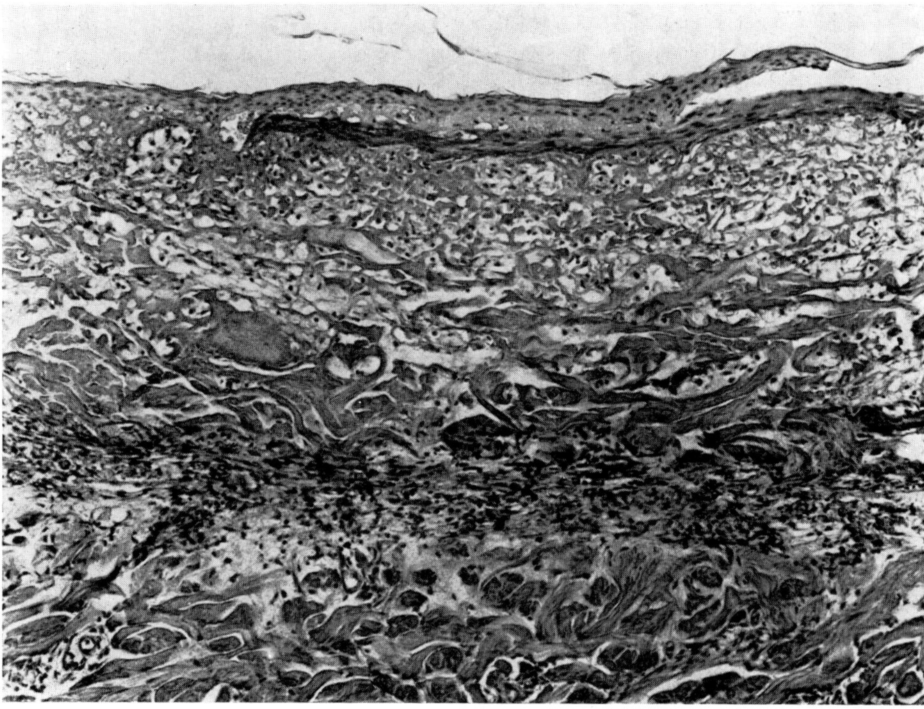

Fig. 1. Epidermis from host migrating under dead epidermis of porcine skin dressing at 7 days. ×200.

epidermis or dressing, had dried. Epidermal migration from the edges of the wound and from hair follicles took place through the dermal collagenous fibrous tissue beneath this scab. It took seven days before the surface was fully covered by new epidermis. Connective tissue regeneration then took place in a fluid layer beneath the new epidermis.

Occlusive dressing

Polythene film prevented dehydration of the wound surface and scab formation and the epidermis migrated across the wound in a film of proteinaceous exudate beneath the dressing. Complete epithelisation took only 3 days. Connective tissue regeneration then took place beneath the new epidermis (10).

Autograft

Migration of epidermis from the cut surfaces of hair follicles was completely inhibited by a fresh autograft. The graft epidermis survived and formed the new permanent epidermal cover. The dermis of the graft was vascularised and fibrous connective tissue formed between the base of the graft and the wound surface. Subsequently the dermal collagen of the graft was lysed and replaced by new connective tissue. Epidermal cysts developed in the graft from surviving epidermal cells of the fragments of hair follicles in the graft.

Fresh allograft

The surface of the graft was invaded by mononuclear cells and the graft epidermis atrophied. Epidermal regeneration took place from the cut surfaces of the hair follicles in the wound, the epidermis migrating through the dermal collagen of the graft below the region of intensive round cell activity, incorporating some of the basal dermal part of the

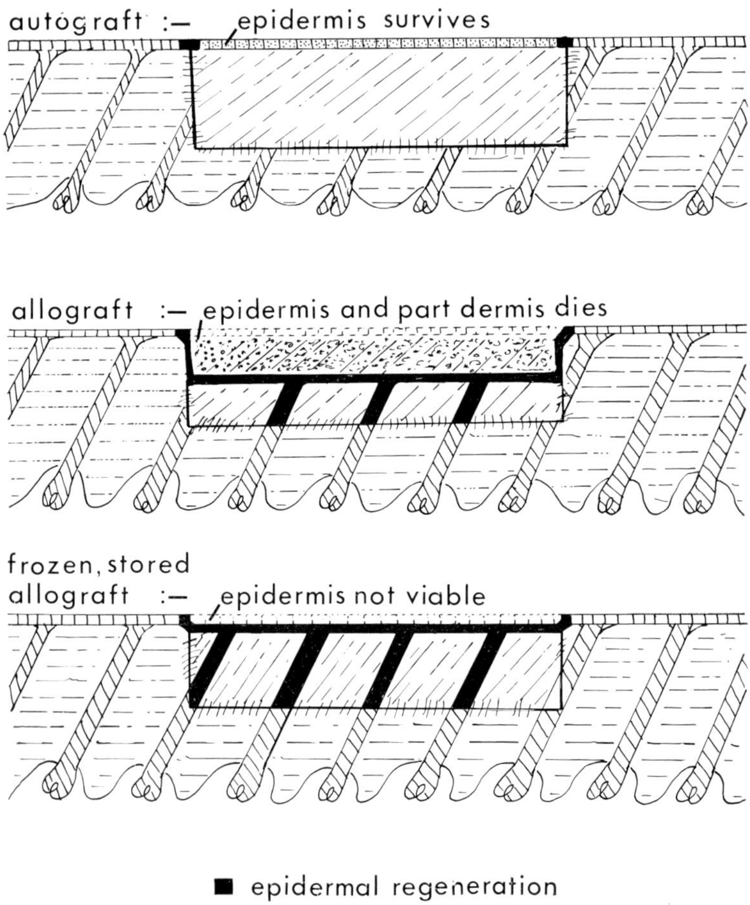

Fig. 2. Epidermal regeneration: autograft, fresh allograft, frozen, stored allograft compared.

graft into the wound. This graft collagen was subsequently lysed and replaced by new connective tissue. Epithelisation was incomplete at 7 days but a continous sheet of epidermis had been established by the tenth day.

Frozen, stored allograft

At the junction of graft-dressing and wound epidermal regeneration from hair follicles had begun, at 3 days, but did not proceed very far. New connective tissue was rapidly formed across the interface. The horny layer of the graftdressing protected the underlying tissue from dehydration and the biological dressing remained moist and supple. Epidermis from the host found its way to the surface of the graft-dressing alongside hair follicles and spread beneath the dead epidermis of the graft-dressing (fig. 1) with the result that the entire dermis of the graft-dressing was incorporated into the wound. A complete new (host) epidermis covered the graft by 14 days. No inflammatory reaction or mononuclear cell invasion took place. The graft-dressing was subsequently lysed and replaced by new connective tissue.

Discussion

Two observations deserve comment: the lack of cellular reaction to the frozen, stored allograft and the different behaviour of the epidermis of the host under different kinds of grafts (fig. 2). Several authors have commented upon the absence or modification of the classical immune response encountered with frozen porcine skin dressings (4, 5, 8, 9).

In these experiments the fresh allografts provoked a marked inflammatory reaction, were invaded by mononuclear cells from the host and the surfaces of the grafts necrosed within about 7 days. They suffered immune rejection.

Frozen, stored allografts provoked none of these cellular reactions. Because a viable epidermis reached the surface of the graft-dressing and survived there and because the graft dermis was invaded by fibroblasts there must have been adequate oxygen and nutrients to support cell life, hence the conditions for cell mediated or humoral immune reactions were satisfied. It appears that the freezing and storing of the pig skin had markedly reduced its antigenicity.

Epidermal regeneration from cell sources in the surface of the wound, separating the graft from its bed took place beneath fresh allografts (through the graft) but not under autografts or frozen stored allografts. The epidermis of the autografts survived, that of the frozen, stored allografts died and was replaced by epidermis from hair follicles in the host — the end result being similar. This behaviour of migrating epidermis is consistent with prior observations (10, 11), namely that epidermis migrates through damaged collagenous tissue but not through healthy connective tissue. The new fibrous tissue rapidly formed across the graft-wound junction, when autografts and frozen, stored allografts were used evidently prevented epidermal migration at this level. This can be construed as further evidence that no damaging immune reaction affected the dermal part of the graft-dressing, at least in the first few days.

These experiments have shown that a porcine skin dressing, used on donor site type wounds on pigs does not function strictly as a dressing in that the dermal component of the graft-dressing is incorporated into the wound. It appears to inhibit the acute cellular inflammatory reactions normally seen under a scab or a synthetic dressing. The keratin of the graft-dressing epidermis provides an adequate water vapour barrier and protects the underlying tissue from dehydration so that the graft-dressing remains moist and supple. The occlusive nature of the dressings promotes rapid healing. Used as an allograft it performs as a biodegradable temporary skin prosthesis, its collagen being gradually replaced by new connective tissue from the host. This work will provide the basis for subsequent studies of xenografts and observations will be made on burns as well as surgical wounds.

Acknowledgements.

I thank D. W. Clarke and S. J. Varley for skillful assistance.

References

1. Baxter, C. R. (1970): Homografts and heterografts as a biological dressing in the treatment of thermal injury. Dept. Surg. Univ. of Texas, U.S.A. Presented at 1st Ann. Congr. Soc. German Plast. Surg. Munich, Sept. 28th, 1970.
2. Bromberg, B. E. (1970): Burn wound management with biologic dressings. N.Y. State J. Med. 70 : 1645.
3. Burleson, R. and Eiseman, B. (1973): Mechanisms of antibacterial effect of biologic dressings. Ann. Surg. 177 : 181.
4. Kelly, A. P. (1972): Cellular immune response to pig skin. Presented at Ann. Meet. Amer. Soc. Plast. Reconstr. Surg. Sept. 1972. Las Vegas, Nevada, U.S.A.
5. Lee, Y. C. (1972): Early heterografting of partial thickness burns. J. Trauma 12 : 818.
6. Miller, T. A., Switzer, W. E., Foley, F. D. and Moncrief, J. A. (1967): Early homografting of second degree burns. Plast. Reconstr. Surg. 40 : 117.
7. Pruitt, B. A. and Silverstein, P. (1971): Methods of resurfacing denuded skin areas. Transpl. Proc. 3 : 1537.
8. Silverstein, P., Warden, G. D., McManus, W. F. and Walker, H. L. (1972): A Study of immune response to split-thickness cutaneous xenograft to improve care of burn wounds in military personnel. Report MEDDH 288 (R1) U.S. Army Inst. Surg. Res., Brooke Army Medical Center, Fort Sam, Houston, Texas, U.S.A.
9. Song, I. C., Bromberg, B. E., Mohn, M. P. and Koehnlein, E. (1966): Heterografts as biological dressings for large skin wounds. Surg. 59 : 576.
10. Winter, G. D. (1972): Epidermal regeneration studied in the domestic pig. In: Epidermal Wound Healing (Maibach, H. E. and Rovee, D. T. eds.). Year Book Medical Publishers, 71.
11. Winter, G. D. (1973): Transcutaneous implants: reactions of the skin-implant interface. Presented at 5th Ann. Biomat. Symp. April 1973. Clemson Univ. S. Carolina, U.S.A. J. Biomed. Mat. Res. (in press).

G. D. W., Royal National Orthopaedic Hosp., Stanmore, Middlesex, Great Britain

TRIAL OF EPIGARD IN THE BURNED PATIENT

A. B. SUTHERLAND

Bangour General Hospital, Broxburn, West Lothian, Great Britain

The search continues for material whether synthetic or biological which can provide temporary cover for extensive areas of skin loss while awaiting availability of donor areas for autograft. Such material should be capable of producing and maintaining healthy granulation tissue while reducing the loss of water, electrolytes and protein from the surface. Epigard is one such material consisting of a reticulated polyurethane foam bonded to an outer film of polypropylene.

Time does not permit discussion of its various uses nor presentation of details of its handling. One case, I hope, presented in detail may bring out some of the points in its use.

A 18 month old boy sustained flame burns of 45 percent of his body surface, about 30 percent being considered full thickness skin loss. Initially the trunk was exposed and the legs dressed with simple absorptive non-impregnated dressings. Loose slough was removed under general anaesthesia on post-burn days 10 and 14.

On day 17 Epigard was applied to the anterior trunk which still showed some adherent slough. At this time, that is on post-burn day 21, the granulations on the left leg were receptive and were autografted. These took well and the trunk dressing with Epigard was continued. On day 28 the Epigard treated area had deteriorated but further application of the material gave improvement, and on day 31 it was considered receptive for autografting. All these grafts took well and grafting was completed with a further small graft, healing being complete by day 50.

In the light of this patient what advantages and/or disadvantages did the material have?

Firstly we felt it did allow us time to recrop donor areas, skin cover being achieved without the use of the posterior trunk as a donor site. This, we felt, would have made nursing difficult with the remaining lesion being anterior. Cover in a burn of this size achieved by post-burn day 50 we feel is adequate and Epigard did not prolong this.

Secondly weight loss was well within our accepted range of 10–15 percent for this extent of burn and age of child. The first rise in weight was noted immediately after the application of Epigard. If this were due to protection offered in terms of evaporative loss it did not appear when intake and output were compared, the insensible loss only becoming less as skin cover was achieved with autograft.

Thirdly this child ran a persistent tachycardia and hyperpyrexia and these do not appear to have been influenced by Epigard application on its own, although perhaps it may have contributed to the improvement which followed the application of skin.

Another child with a similar injury did, in fact, show quite dramatic improvement in a hyperpyrexia and tachycardia with no other change in treatment other than the application of Epigard.

This material although still in an experimental stage would appear to be useful when used in this way in the local care of the patient with the more extensive injury.

A. B. S., Bangour General Hospital,
Broxburn, West Lothian, Great Britain

SYNKRYT (SYNCOVER) — SYNTHETIC GRAFT*

J. SAMOHÝL, D. IMRIŠOVÁ, S. MARYŠKA, O. SAMOHÝLOVÁ and M. KRÁČMER

Department of Plastic Surgery, J. E. Purkyně University, Brno, National Textile Research Institute, Liberec, Department for Research and Application of Ionising Radiation, Brno, Department of Surgery, Military Hospital, Brno, and Third Department of Surgery, J. E. Purkyně University, Brno, Czechoslovakia

In treating deep burns, it is often necessary to temporarily cover large skin defects to prevent infection of the exposed structures and to reduce loss of body fluids.

At present, either homografts or pig heterografts are used for this purpose. However, it often happens that both of them are not easily available in the required, relatively large quantities. In addition, they provoke immunological response and their quality varies.

For these reasons, some institutes in the world started to develop a synthetic substitute for skin grafts.

Reports on these experiments and especially some papers read at the Second World Burn Congress in Prague have inspired our team of the Department of Plastic Surgery in Brno and the Liberec Textile Research Institute's Department for Research and Application of Ionising Radiation in Brno to co-operate and to develop a synthetic skin cover, which is now called Synkryt (Syncover — synthetic cover).

It consists of two layers: the inferior, corresponding to the corium, 3 mm thick and fairly porous, is made of a special type of polyurethane; it is this layer which will be directly applied to the wound. The upper layer, corresponding to the epidermis, is thin, with standard permeability, less pronounced than in the inferior layer. This upper layer consists of acrylate on a textile net (Fig. 1).

Synkryt is available in various sizes, sterilized by radiation, packed in transparent plastic foil securing long-term sterility (Fig. 2).

When applied to the wound, Synkryt — whether dry or wet — adheres well to the surface. The wound secretion is in this case absorbed by the spongy polyurethane and leucocyte mass. Thanks to the permeability of the upper layer of Synkryt, the wound does not dry up or get macerated. There are no signs of irritation of the surface. Synkryt seems — in a way — to conserve the wound secretion.

Blood vessels may penetrate into Synkryt in the course of time, but not farther than into the lowest layer.

If applied to a sterile wound, Synkryt can be left in place for days or even weeks. The covered defect remains fresh, prepared for final grafting.

* Dedicated to Professor Karfík on the occasion of the 70th anniversary of his birthday.

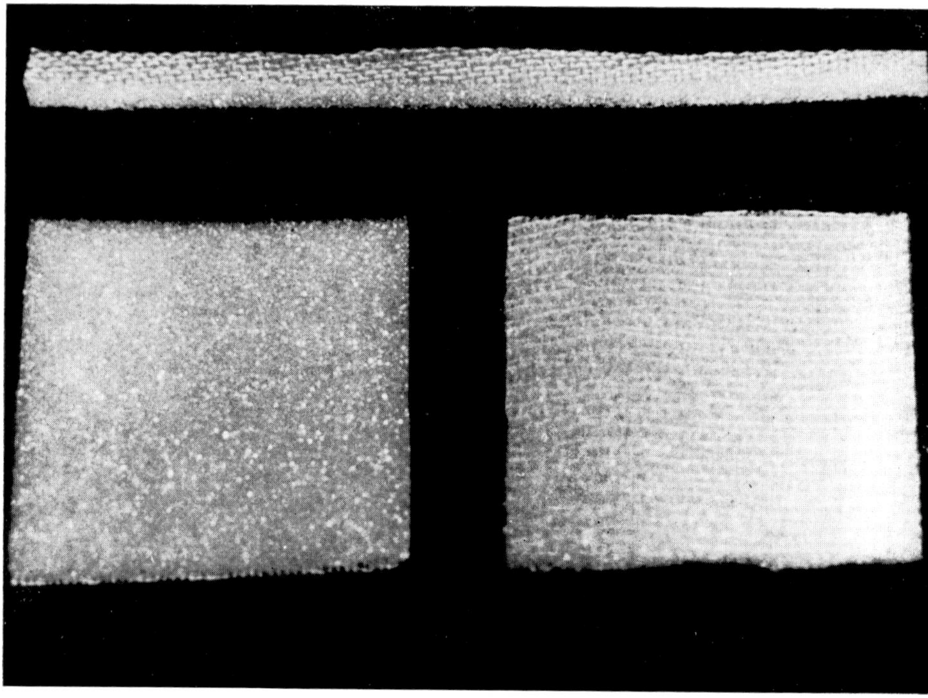

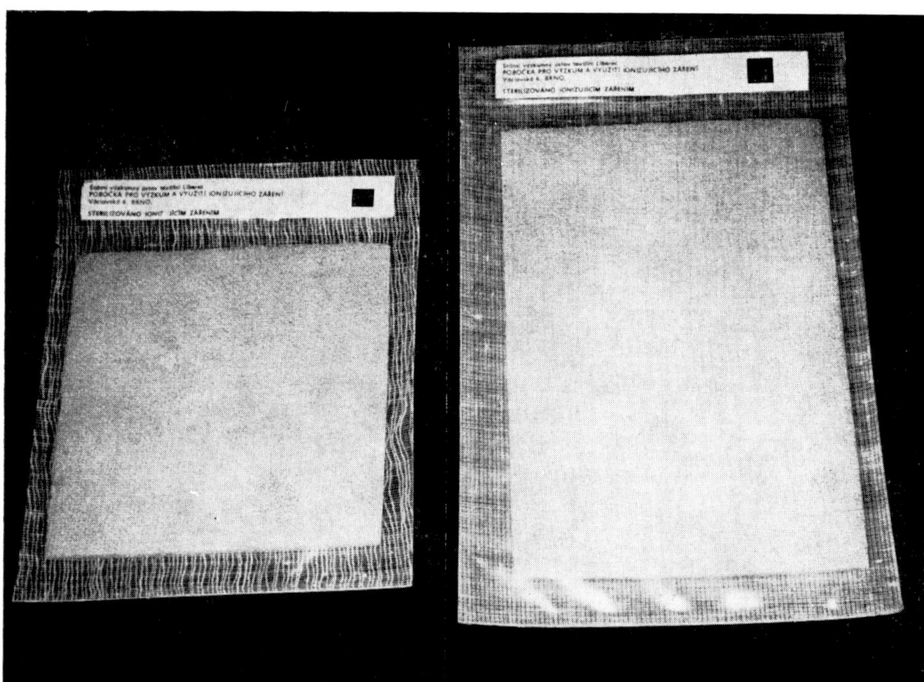

← *Fig. 1.* Synkryt — both sides and cross-section.

Synkryt may be applied without additional dressing; more often, however, the dressing is supplemented by gauze and bandage, especially in wounds with abundant secretion, which is absorbed by gauze.

After the completion of experiments with Synkryt on animals, clinical testing was started at the Department of Plastic Surgery, the Military Hospital and the 3rd Surgical

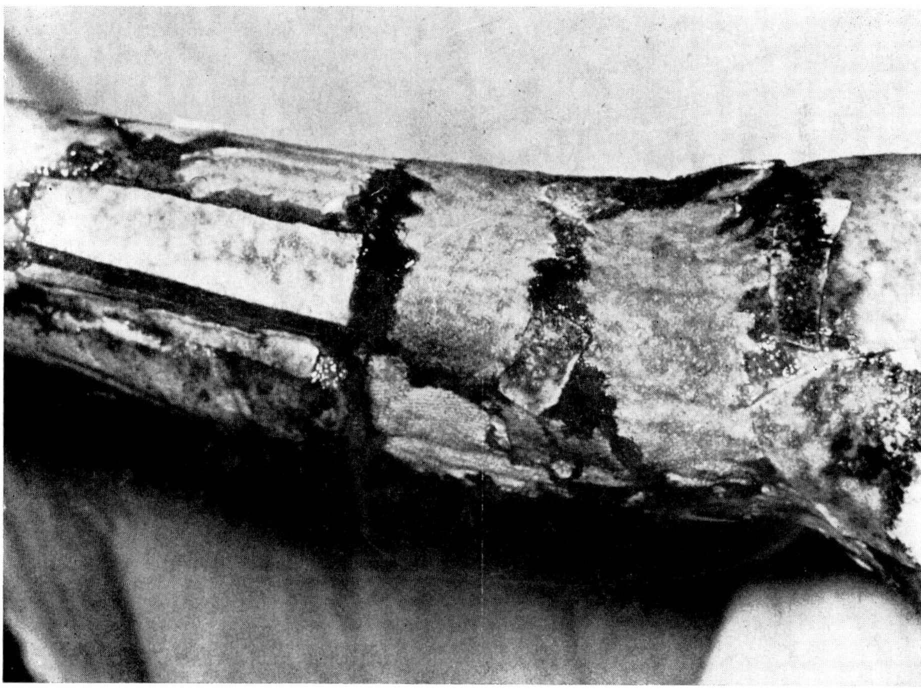

Fig. 3. Large chronic traumatic skin defect of the leg. Owing to the patient's bad general condition, only a part was covered with autografts; the rest was covered with Synkryt for 8 days.

Clinic — all three of them in Brno; at present, futher clinical testing is carried on by other departments, among them by the Burn Units in Prague and Ostrava.

We have based the Synkryt indications upon our first clinical trials:

1. Synkryt is useful in covering fresh skin defects when autografts are not available. Synkryt is either applied or fastened with stitches. In a few days it is replaced by a graft.

2. Synkryt is suitable for covering granulating skin defects when autografts are not available or when the surgeon decided against them. Strips of Synkryt are gradually

← *Fig. 2.* Sterile packages of Synkryt.

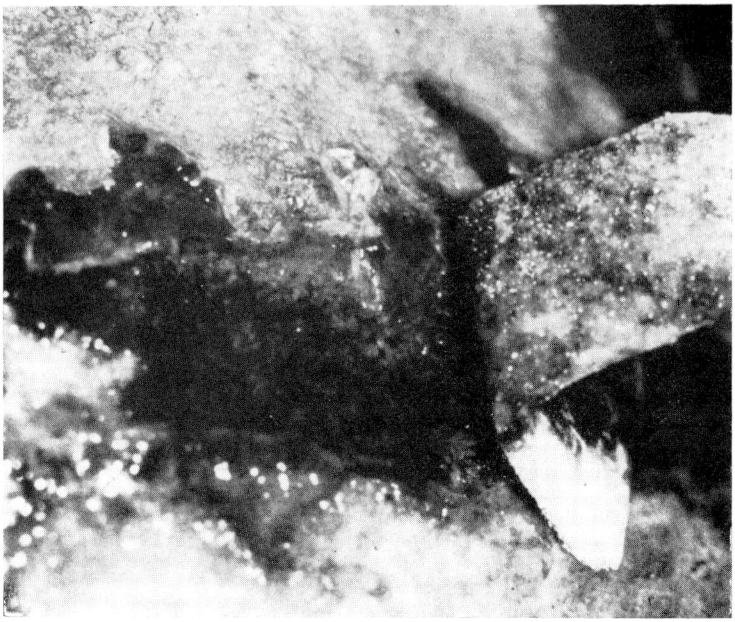

Fig. 4. Detail view of the wound shown in Fig. 3: Synkryt was removed, the raw surface is clean and ready for autograft.

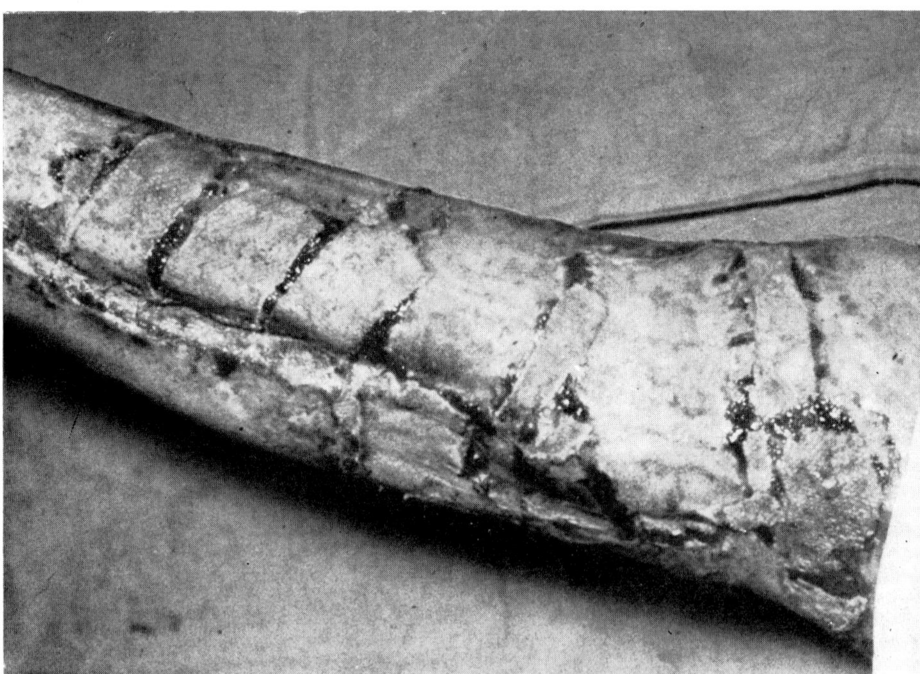

Fig. 5. First dressing after autografts replaced Synkryt. All grafts took excellently.

replaced by autografts. Our clinical experience has shown that Synkryt can replace the skin for a period of a week, a fortnight or even longer. There is some capillary bleeding when Synkryt is removed after a longer period (Fig. 3, 4, 5).

Synkryt cannot fulfill its graft function well if applied to weak granulations where even autograft would not take. However, it can even under such circumstances influence the quality of granulating tissue favourably, provided that Synkryt dressing is changed more frequently, that the wound is cleaned and eventually covered with antibiotic-soaked Synkryt. In this way, Synkryt acts as a dressing; this is of advantage especially in chronic granulating leg sores where we get modified sponge dressing.

3. Synkryt is useful for covering surgical sutures. All these indications are continually tested. Interestingly enough, Synkryt did not prove suitable for covering donor sites; on the other hand, it was successful in 2nd degree burns. The Synkryt structure may be possibly a little changed in the future.

According to our experience, Synkryt has proved to be an ever ready wound-cover for surgical purposes, easily available in any quantity and size wanted; it can be easily stored and its sterility is not endangered. It can be universally used and no immunological response is to be feared.

J. S., Dept. of Plastic Surgery,
Berkova 34–38,
612 00 Brno 12, Czechoslovakia

THE USE OF XENOGRAFTS AS TEMPORARY COVERAGE ON MESH GRAFTS IN EXTENSIVE BURNS

H. BOHMERT

Division of Plastic Surgery, Department of Surgery, University of Munich, F.R.G.

In spite of acknowledged advantages for accomplishing early closure of extensive burn wounds using mesh grafts, the value of this method is limited by various disadvantages, such as continued loss of biological fluids, the lack of control of infection, and the potential cosmetic disfigurement. This led us to consider whether these disadvantages could be overcome by covering the area of mesh grafts with a suitable material.

On the basis of preliminary investigations we decided that, for mechanical, biological and immunological reasons, fetal calf skin constitutes a suitable covering material. As also observed by other investigators (2, 3, 5) fetal calf skin suppresses inflammatory reactions and induces the development of a healthy highly vascularsized granulating tissue. It has been noted that there is a surprising lack of host reaction to these grafts. The process of epithelialisation has continued extremely satisfactorily underneath them, with a marked reduction in infection of the burn wounds, decrease of exudative protein loss, and the control of evaporative water loss. Considering these advantages, the idea was to evaluate whether these xenograft material would become firmly adherent to the graft bed on top of the mesh grafts with their open spaces in order to accomplish earlier complete closure of the burn wound.

Experimental investigations

Experimentally, three raw areas of ten centimeters in diameter created on the backs of each of twelve dwarf pigs were covered first by mesh grafts and then either by fetal calf skin — pretreated with nucleic acids to act as an immunosuppressive agent as earlier described by the author (1, 4) with collagen or moist saline dressings. The mesh grafted defects covered with the fetal calf skin showed distinctly better healing than with any other method. There was no destruction of the mesh graft and the level of the granulations was even and flat. This temporary covering remained firmly adherent until the entire area beneath was covered with epithelium, at an average time of 8 days. With collagen sheets, the defects were epithelialised 1–2 days earlier, but contraction of the defect was appreciable. When wet dressings were used as covering material, partial loss of the mesh grafts was observed and a very pronounced wound contraction became obvious. Total epithelialisation took 10–12 days.

Clinical experience

In an attempt to evaluate clinically the use of fetal calf skin, pretreated as described, as a possible healing adjuvant on mesh grafts, we applied this material to twenty-seven patients with large burn wounds. The results confirmed the animal experiments. Infection was reduced and wound healing was accelerated. The immediate elimination of fever was dramatic and psychological improvement usually noted. In addition, pain was reduced and the patients' general condition became earlier improved once fetal calf skin had been applied on the meshed grafts. The conversion of the open into a closed wound at this earlier stage may be responsible for the great improvement. The technique and clinical progress in one patient with extensive third degree burns is illustrated by slides.

The combination of mesh grafts with these xenografts as a temporary coverage has proved to be remarkably useful in reducing and preventing infection and decreasing fluid loss. Healing is noticeably better beneath them, and its application stimulates markedly the growth of healthy, highly vascular granulation tissue, and thus encourages maximum take of the mesh grafts. It is apparent that the application of these xenografts serves not only as a stimulatory substance but also accelerates epithelialisation. Total epithelialisation of the interstices between the ribbons of the mesh graft was achieved between the 5th and 7th postoperative days in contrast to the usual time of between 9 and 12 days. The final appearence was improved cosmetically, and compared favourably to the use of sheet grafts. Scar formation and postoperative contraction were noticeably decreased.

References

1. Ashley, F. L., McNall, E. G., Dutt, N. R., Garcia, E. N. and Sloan, R. F. (1960): The effects of nucleic acids tolerance. Ann. N.Y. Acad. Sci. 87: 429.
2. Bohmert, H., Sollinger, H. W., Seinfeld, H. und Brendel, W. (1971): Deckung ausgedehnter Wundflächen durch Kombination von autogenen Netztransplantaten und fetalen Hautxenotransplantaten. Chir. plast. 1: 72.
3. Rogers, B. O. and Converse, J. M. (1958): Bovine embryo zoografts as temporary biological dressing for burns and other skin defects. Plast. reconstruct. Surg. 22 : 471.
4. Seinfeld, H., Brendel, W. and Bohmert, H. (1971): Nucleic acids as immunosuppressive adjuvant in xenogeneic grafts for extensive burns. Transactions of the Fifth Internat. Congr. of Plast. reconstr. Surg. Sydney. Butterworth, 717.
5. Sokolic, I. H., Farpour, A., Ulin, A. W. and Howard, J. (1959): The use of the heterograft skin as a biological dressing. Surg. Forum 10 : 847.

Priv. Doz. Dr. H.B.,
Abteilung für Plastische Chirurgie,
Chirurgische Universitätsklinik München,
Thalkirchner Str. 48,
BRD — 8000 München 2, F.R.G.

CHANGES IN EVAPORATIVE WATER LOSS AND HYPERMETABOLISM IN BURNED PATIENTS AFTER APPLICATION OF XENOGRAFTS

G. ARTURSON

Burn Center, University Hospital, Uppsala, Sweden

The increased evaporation following thermal injury causes an increased evaporative heat loss. It is widely accepted that in compensation for this heat loss the burned patient's heat production is increased. If this hypothesis is correct blockage of the evaporative heat loss should result in a concurrent reduction in metabolic rate.

In the present investigation the hypothesis that increased evaporative heat loss is a major cause of hypermetabolism in burns was tested. This was done by reducing evaporative water loss in patients with burns using lyophilized porcine skin xenografts as a topical burn therapy and observing the effect on the metabolic rate.

Material and Methods

In a series of patients with burns varying from 30 to 70 percent of the body surface area the following measurements were made before and at different times after application of porcine skin xenografts: insensible weight loss, local evaporative water loss, heat loss by radiation, oxygen consumption and carbon dioxide production.

None of the patients had subnormal rectal temperature when exposed and no patients were shivering. All patients were treated similarly with plasma, albumin, Ringer's bicarbonate solutions, fat emulsions and amino acids. The ambient temperature and relative humidity was kept constant.

Results

The results showed that the fluid loss by evaporation in the patients was of the magnitude of 20–40 mg $cm^{-2}h^{-1}$. This loss was about the same in the temperature range between 25 and 35 degrees of centigrade at constant relative humidity of about 20 percent. By topical control of water loss with porcine skin xenografts during three consecutive days the evaporation was reduced by 80–90 percent (Table I and Fig. 1).

By this treatment it was, however, not possible to reduce the increased oxygen consumption significantly, in other words the metabolic rate which was increased by 60–70 percent in the burned patients was not changed after application of xenografts (Fig. 1). This was at least partly due to the fact that blockage of evaporative heat loss resulted in a moderate

TABLE I.

Evaporative water loss in mg cm^{-2}h^{-1} $\pm$ S.E. normal skin and from different degrees of burnt skin before and on different times after application of lyophilized porcine skin xenografts (n — number of measurements)

Type of area measured	n	*Application of xenografts*	
		Before	*After*
Normal skin	10	1.1 $\pm$ 0.4 mg cm^{-2}h^{-1}	—
Second degree burn	11	34.6 $\pm$ 3.5 mg cm^{-2}h^{-1}	6.9 $\pm$ 2.4 mg cm^{-2}h^{-1}
Third degree burn	13	24.4 $\pm$ 2.1 mg cm^{-2}h^{-1}	2.4 $\pm$ 1.1 mg cm^{-2}h^{-1}

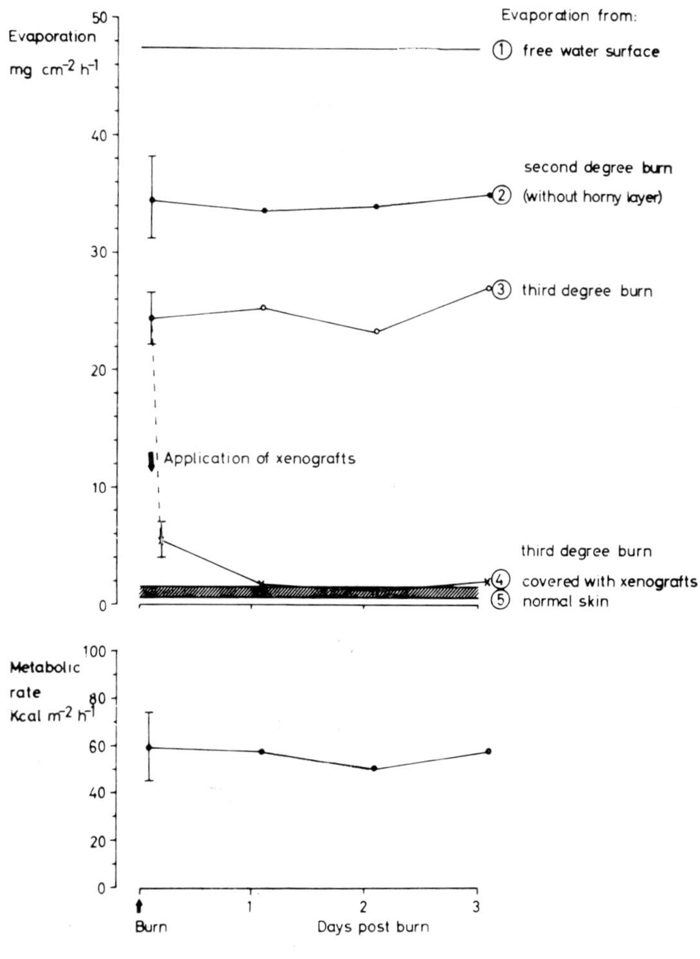

Fig. 1. Upper part: The evaporation from second and third degree burns with and without application of lyophilized porcine skin xenografts compared with the evaporation from free water surface and normal skin. — Lower part: The metabolic rate of patients with burns covered with xenografts. Mean values and $\pm$ S.E. (vertical bars) from six adult patients with burns varying from 30 to 70 percent of the body surface area.

increase in body temperature which increased heat loss by the three remaining routes, radiation, conduction and convection. As a rule the surface temperature of the xenografts applied on the burnt surface was found to be about 0.5–1.0 degrees of centigrade higher than on the normal skin and 2–3 degrees of centigrade higher than on the open burned wound.

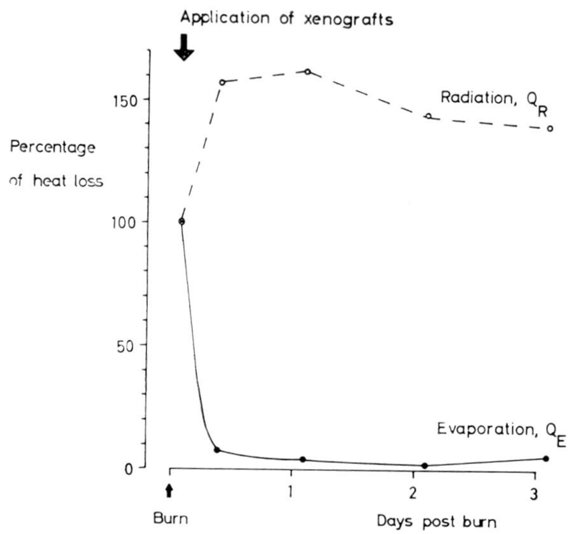

Fig. 2. Percentage of heat loss from six adult patients with burns after application of lyophilized porcine skin xenografts. The heat loss from radiation is increased concomitant with the decrease in evaporative heat loss.

According to the Stefan-Boltzmann law the heat loss from radiation increased concomitant with the decrease in evaporative heat loss after application of xenografts (Fig. 2).

Discussion

In the present investigation a 72-hour reduction of evaporation, a major route of heat loss, did not reduce heat production significantly. This is in accordance with similar results by Zawacki *et al.* (9) and suggests several things:

The relationship between evaporative cooling and metabolic rate in the burned patient is not as clearly defined as has been concluded from previous studies. Topical burn therapy which decreases evaporative water loss does not necessarily as a consequence reduce the metabolic rate.

The increase in metabolic rate, the hypermetabolism, thus seems to be primarily stimulated by mechanisms other than (1) evaporative cooling (6, 8). Several other different mechanisms are possible:

2. prolonged increases of catecholamine excretion may be partly responsible for the hypermetabolism (4). Already six years ago Harrison and co-workers demonstrated a significant correlation between the magnitude of oxygen consumption increase and the degree to which catecholamine excretion is elevated in thermal burns;

3. varying degree of sepsis and pain both of which tend to elevate the heat production (9);
4. although there is no evidence in previous literature of thyroid hyperactivity following burn injury this possibility cannot be ruled out (3). Since then investigations of thyroid physiology has proved a fertile field of research and there has been much progress in the development of techniques for measuring free thyroid hormones, which might play an important role in post-injury metabolism;
5. for the present discussion it is also of interest that infusion of amino acids has a similar effect to that observed in hyperthyroidism (7);
6. the possibility that injury or sepsis may produce uncoupling of oxidation and phosphorylation (2) might be another attractive hypothesis but remains to be documented;
7. finally, part of the increases in caloric expenditure might be related to the processes of hepatic gluconeogenesis and urea synthesis (5). Therefore it is of importance to examine not only the mechanisms for the production of new glucose but also the mechanisms for mobilizing and oxidizing fatty acids since they represent the major source of calories in patients with burns.

Summary

In the present investigation the following hypothesis was tested: Is the increased evaporative heat loss a major cause of hypermetabolism in burns? This was done by reducing evaporative water loss using lyophilized porcine skin xenografts as a topical burn therapy during three consecutive days and observing the effect on the metabolic rate. The results showed that this treatment reduced the evaporative water loss by 80–90 percent but no significant change was found in the elevated metabolic rate. This indicates that the increased metabolic rate in major burns is primarily stimulated by mechanisms other than evaporative cooling. Several other possibilities have been discussed and are of importance to take into account for future research. It is of special importance as several modern investigations indicate that the caloric loss in extensive burns exceeds the compensatory capability of the body and thereby constitute a major factor in the pathogenesis of burn death. This fact also explains why so many interesting therapeutical attempts are going on trying to reduce the heat loss in thermal trauma.

References

1. Arturson, G. (1971): Evaporation and fluid replacement. In: Research in Burns, H. Huber, Bern-Shethpart-Wien, 520.
2. Caswell, A. H. (1969): Proton permeability and the regulation of potassium permeability in mitochondria by uncoupling agents. J. Membrane Biol. 1 : 53.
3. Cope, O., Nardi, G. L., Quisano, M., Rorit, R. L., Stanbury, J. B. and Wright, A. (1953): Metabolic rate and thyroid function following acute thermal trauma in man. Ann. Surg. 137 : 165.
4. Harrison, T. S., Seaton, J. F. and Feller, I. (1967): Relationship of increased oxygen consumption to catecholamine excretion in thermal burns. Ann. Surg. 165 : 169.
5. Kinney, J. M., Gump, F. E. and Long, C. L. (1973): Energy and tissue fuel in human injury and sepsis. In: Adv. exp. Med. Biol. 33 : 401.
6. Lieberman, Z. H. and Lansche, J. M. (1956): Effects of thermal injury on metabolic rate and insensible water loss in the rat. Surg. Forum 7 : 83.
7. Myers, J. D. (1954): In: Shock and Circulatory Homeostasis. Madison Printing Co. Inc., Madison, New Jersey.
8. Roe, C. F., Kinney, J. M. and Blair, C. (1964): Water and heat exchange in third-degree burns. Surgery 56 : 212.
9. Zawacki, B. E., Spitzer, K. W., Mason Jr., A. D. and Johns, L. A. (1970): Does increased evaporative water loss cause hypermetabolism in burned patients? Ann. Surg. 171 : 236.

G. A., Burn Center, University Hospital
S-750 14 Uppsala, Sweden

PRIMARY EXCISION OF FULL THICKNESS BURNS UP TO 40 P.C. OF BODY SURFACE FOLLOWED IMMEDIATELY BY MICRO- OR MESHGRAFTS

R. P. HERMANS

The Red Cross Hospital, Beverwijk, The Netherlands

It is now nearly three years ago that in this wonderful city I had the honour of speaking at the meeting of the I.S.B.I. about primary excision of large full thickness burns followed immediately by mesh- or micrografting. At that time I was one of the very few who advocated early excision of extensive full thickness burns and I feel very happy that in these past three years the picture has changed substantially. In many distinguished burn centers, excision of these burns has become more and more the treatment of choice.

I think I do not have to talk extensively about the adventages of early excision, let me just summarize them:

1. The necrotic tissue is the main basis and entrance for infection, it should therefore be removed as soon as possible.
2. Early excision and immediate grafting shortens healing and hospitalisation time considerably.
3. With this treatment many contractures can be prevented.
4. Return of sensation — a much neglected subject — is much better.
5. The general condition of the patient stays better.

Early excision of extensive full thickness burns puts us before two important problems:

1. Large excisions are major surgical procedures; they intensify the problem of post burn shock. My colleague Dr. Spijker is going to talk about the special reanimation problems connected with these procedures. The surgeon can try to help by preventing blood loss by taking the following precautions:
   a) Several teams should work on the patient at the same time so as to shorten operation time.
   b) During the excision the limbs concerned should be suspended in the vertical position.
   c) Blood loss is much less if the skin is more or less pulled off instead of actually excised.
   d) We restrain from the tourniquet method as we have observed that after taking the tourniquet much bleeding occurs, endangering the grafts.
2. How to cover the large excised areas. Since 1965 we have been using spreading techniques. Originally we used the Meek micrografts giving an enlargement of 9 times the

donor size. Unfortunately the factory does not make the prefolded bandages anymore, so we had to switch over to mesh grafts. We now use the Tanner machine, and lately more and more the Drapier machine of which the latter one is relatively unknown, yet so very handy.

Handling the mesh grafts has become very much easier since my assistant Dr. Kreis suggested spraying the donor area with a thin layer of plastic before taking off the skin.

Our procedure is as follows:

The excision is done as soon as the general condition of the patient tolerates the operation, preferably before the fourth postburn day.

One team of surgeons pulls off the skin while another team prepares the meshed skin, putting it on the denuded area as soon as possible.

The grafted areas are covered with one layer of tulle gras, then fine mesh gauze, then synthetic cotton wool and an elastic bandage.

The bandages are changed every 5 days. After 15 to 20 days the meshed skin usually has grown out very rapidly in such a way that the originally large full thickness area is reduced to a very much smaller size, thus converting the extensive burn into a small burn within three weeks.

In the beginning we had hoped to cover all the full thickness areas in one sitting; it has turned out that small defects remain, necessitating secondary procedures.

If there wos infection we used silversulfadiazine or silver nitrate on the meshgrafts. Very lately we have been experimenting with covering the mesh grafts with porcine skin; so far we have not seen any benefit from this.

Indication for primary excision and immediate mesh- or micrografting are:

1. Full thickness burns of areas between 10 an 40 percent of body surface.
2. Full thickness burns of smaller areas if the patient also has extensive partial thickness burns thus limiting the possibility of taking autografts.
3. Smaller full thickness burns in the extremely old or young with the idea of having to take off less skin and so keeping the operation less traumatic.

Results

So far we have treated 41 patient. 8 of these patients died. Only two of the patients that died had burns smaller than 60 percent of body surface. One of these two died of cerebromeningitis following severe cranial injury, the other patient had carbonisation of the face, she died of cerebral edema. Summarising this form of therapy we believe that in many aspects the results are much better than with conservative therapy while we did not find any increase in mortality.

Dr. R.P.H., Zeestraat 129,
Beverwijk, The Netherlands

CLINICAL EXPERIENCE WITH CHORION-AMNION GRAFTS USED AS BIOLOGICAL DRESSING

Š. ŠIMKO, R. KLEN and J. BABÍK

Burns Unit, Košice-Šaca, and Tissue Bank, Faculty Hospital, Regional National Health Institute in Hradec Králové, Czechoslovakia

The deeper our insight into the treatment of burn shock, the more emphasis must be placed on the need of a suitable biological dressing for burn wounds. In our department, we investigated the use of various biological materials, among them lyophilised chorion-amnion grafts supplied by the Tissue Bank, Faculty Hospital, Regional National Health Institute in Hradec Králové (1).

We used 256 stored chorion-amnion tissues in 35 thermally burned patients. In selecting our patients we considered their general condition, the appearance and state of burned areas and the possibility of covering them with skin autografts or homografts. The patients' age ranged from one to 81 years. Thirty patients had 2nd and 3rd degree burns extending up to 79 per cent of their total body surface. In 15 cases, chorion-amnion grafts were used for granulating surfaces, in 10 cases we covered with them fresh surfaces after necrectomy.

We expected the formation of a surface suitable for autografting, while in minor burns, smaller in extent and lesser in degree, we anticipated integral healing. We kept a check on microbial flora and on pH. In five cases the grafts were applied to fresh donor sites.

After rehydration for 10 minutes in a solution of Ringer's lactate (Hartmann), the rehydrated tissue on tylexol was applied to the prepared surface. In cases of fresh burns, preparations included necrectomy, while granulating surfaces were washed with hexachlorphenolic soap and water.

Most frequently, i.e. fifteen times, chorion-amnion grafts were used to cover granulations, ten times they were applied to fresh surfaces after necrectomy. In five cases we used them for the treatment of chronic postburn defects (in one woman patient we treated a two-year old defect).

After removing the tylexol, we applied the rehydrated grafts in the open treatment method, using either a tent or a Vikers air-bubble. Limbs with extensive circular burn injuries were placed on an extension (Kirschner). Grafts were maintained for 3 to 5 days. When no firm adhesion to the base occurred (air-bubble, serous exudate, haematoma), the grafts disintegrated within 24 hours and were replaced by new ones. Graft application was never repeated more than four times in the same patient. The removal of firmly adhering dry chorion-amnion grafts helped to remove the remaining necrotic tissues. The base appeared as a viable surface with capillary bleeding, suitable for a skin autograft cover. The application of chorion-amnion grafts in the closed tratment method was unsuccessful, the grafts being always washed away.

Donor sites were also successfully covered with these grafts, healing without defects within 10 to 12 days. The chorion-amnion grafts dry up and slough off spontaneously. When chorion-amnion grafts were used to cover infested granulations, the infection was in most cases arrested. So far, little is known about the mechanism of this effect. We believe that the grafts: a) act as a barrier against infection from outside; b) reduce acidity; c) improve phagocytosis and reduce exudation by raising the temperature of underlying tissues.

Chorion-amnion grafts adhere to the burn-wound by fibroelastic bonds, thus mechanically preventing accumulation of pus — and this is of greatest importance in our struggle against spreading infection. When chorion-amnion grafts were applied to minor burns, both in extent and depth, the results confirmed our expectations: there followed complete healing under the graft due to epithalisation from the wound edges and from the epithelium remaining around glands and follicles.

Even after repeated chorion applications we found neither local nor general reactions. The patients' condition improved, pain was reduced and we noticed local disappearance of infection and an improved surface.

In conclusion, we may say that chorion-amnion grafts are suitable: a) for covering surfaces without necroses, if applied in the open treatment method and not left in place for more than 5 days; b) for preparing surfaces for autografting; c) for covering donor sites.

Reference

KLEN, R. (1971): Preparation of chorion and/or amnion grafts used in burns. In: Research in Burns. H. Huber Verlag, Bern, 235.

Š.Š., ZÚNZ VSŽ,
044 53 Košice-Šaca, Czechoslovakia

ENZYMATIC DEBRIDEMENT OF BURN NECROSIS

J. MOSEROVÁ, Z. KONÍČKOVÁ, E. BĚHOUNKOVÁ, R. VRABEC, J. BLÁHA and A. LETTL

Burns Unit, Charles University, Prague, Czechoslovakia

In experiments carried out on laboratory pigs, the authors tested the possibility of debriding thermally damaged skin by the enzyme Collagenase, product of the Institute of Sera and Vaccines (SEVAC) Prague. The crude enzyme collagenase was obtained from Clostridium histolyticum No. 3253 cultures. The effect of the enzyme applied locally was tested both on burned and unburned skin.

28 adult laboratory pigs weighing 25–30 kg were used in the experiments. Collagenase was applied in different unguentous vehicles on burned skin, decorticated and intact skin. The unguent without enzyme was applied on control areas in corresponding anatomical localizations. Standard non-contact burns (full-thickness in the centre, partial thickness on the periphery) were produced by a special apparatus. The unguent was applied immediately following injury (burning and decortication) in a 2–3 mm thick layer, covered by dry gauze and left in place for 24 hours. After 24 hours, dressings were removed and the softened necrotic tissue was wiped off. Results were evaluated macroscopically and samples were taken for histological examination.

The lytic effect of Collagenase, concentrations ranging from 0.5 to 2.0 per cent, was tested in 12 different unguentous vehicles. The effect of Collagenase SEVAC was also compared with the effect of Iruxol (Knoll), a product which also contains collagenase.

With the majority of unguentous vehicles used, 1 per cent concentration of the enzyme sufficed to insure the desintegration of thermally damaged skin within 24 hours (Iruxol was markedly less effective).

No macroscopic changes were observed on decorticated skin after local tratment with Collagenase. Only slight, superficial changes of some collagen fibres were observed microscopically. These appeared to be due to superficial collagen destruction caused by decortication. Intact skin treated by the enzyme for 24 hours was found unchanged both microscopically and histologically. No changes were found on the controls either.

At present, more experiments are being carried out, in which the authors study the healing process of excised 3rd degree burns, burns treated by Collagenase, and burns in which the necrosis is allowed to slough off spontaneously. Transplantation possibilities and results are also being tested.

The enzymatic product we used in our experiments was called Debridin and was recently passed for clinical trials. Debridin contains not only Collagenase, but also non-specific proteases. The unguentous vehicle chosen for clinical trials ensures the possibility to store the product at 4 degrees of centigrade for long periods of time or for shorter periods of time at room temperature, without loss of enzymatic activity.

At the Prague Burn Centre, Debridin was applied up to now to 12 patients with full-thickness burns, on a limited area (0.5–1.0 per cent body surface area) within 2–7th day following injury. In all cases, repeated application of the enzyme proved to be necessary (the enzyme had to be applied for 24 hours 2–5 times). The number of 24-hour treatments was lowered by previous application of dressings soaked in Aserbine. The lytic effect of Debridin was expressed in disintegration of thermally damaged tissues which could be wiped off, similarly as in animal experiments.

The lytic effect of Debridin in clinical trials appears to be less marked than in experiments on laboratory pigs. Nevertheless, the results are quite encouraging. It should be stressed, that in experiments, the enzyme was applied immediately following injury, while in clinical trials it could only be applied after some lapse of time on necrotic tissues in a higher degree of dehydration.

Both by experimental and clinical results, it was proved, that Debridin had a highly selective lytic effect on thermally damaged collagen, while it does not attack intact tissues. Debridin may be of considerable value especially in the debridement of burns in patients, where surgery and anesthesia are contraindicated as well as in cleansing the base of defects from residual necrotic tissues after spontaneous or surgical debridement.

J. M., Burns Unit,
Legerova 63,
120 00 Praha 2, Czechoslovakia

EXPERIENCE FROM FIVE-YEAR USE OF EARLY SURGERY IN DEEP BURNS

I. PEDIŠIĆ

Mother and Child Welfare Institute, Department of Pediatric Surgery, Zagreb, Yugoslavia

In the last five years, 1426 children with burns have been hospitalized at the Ward for Burns of the Mother and Child Welfare Institute's Department of Pediatric Surgery in Zagreb. Early surgery (tangential excision of necrotic tissue and immediate skin grafting) carried out 2–5 days after the accident has been applied in 482 cases of deep burns. In this work we have taken advantage of the great experience of the pioneer of the method. Z. Janžekovič from Maribor, and the works of Jackson and Stone, Lawrence and Groves, and others.

Clinical Diagnosis of the Depth of Burns

Since in our cases most patients are under 4 years of age, analgesia is of little use for indicating the depth of the burn because co-operation with such young patients in this respect is almost impossible. Examination by analysing the effects of pressure has proved of greater use, and so has also a detailed inquiry into the cause of the burns since we know that, for instance, fire, electric current, and glowing objects invariably produce deep lesions. The outward appearance of the burn on admission and also during primary treatment and at each dressing (carried out every day) can help a great deal in the assesment of the depth of the burn.

According to our experience, a white, smooth surface without secretion (which is seen after removing blisters) as long as 24 or 48 hours after the accident, as well as a reddish-brown surface not turning pale on pressure are also indicators of a deep burn. Dark-yellow to dark-brown surfaces may with certainty be regarded as a safe sign of deep burns. However, a safe early diagnosis can be made only on the operating table by applying thin tangential cuts with the Blair knife. Dead tissue is distinguished from live one by spotted bleeding and the colour. By gradually applying ever deeper cuts all non-bleeding areas and all the areas with thrombosed vessels are cut away. Attention should be paid not to cut deeper than necessary so as to preserve, if possible, deeper dermal layers. Of course, if it proves necessary, cuts go deeper into the subdermal tissue, removing indistinctly reddish fatty parts.

Immediately after this early necrectomy — applied in all deep dermal and full thickness burns — is completed, the defects are autografted after Thiersch by arranging the grafts to reach the edge of the healthy tissue but not quite touch it (so as to avoid scars on the edges). A compressive bandage is then applied and immobilization is achieved by iron wool pads. If there are not enough autografts, homografts are used, but efforts must be

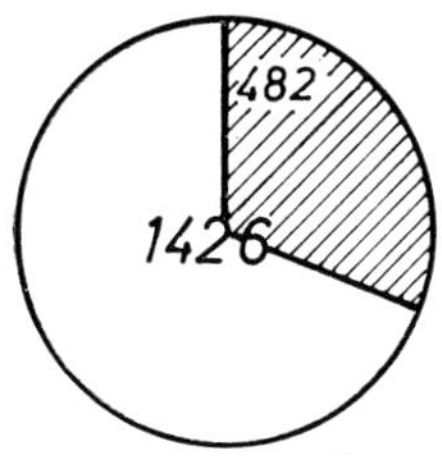

Nº of patients and performed necrect.

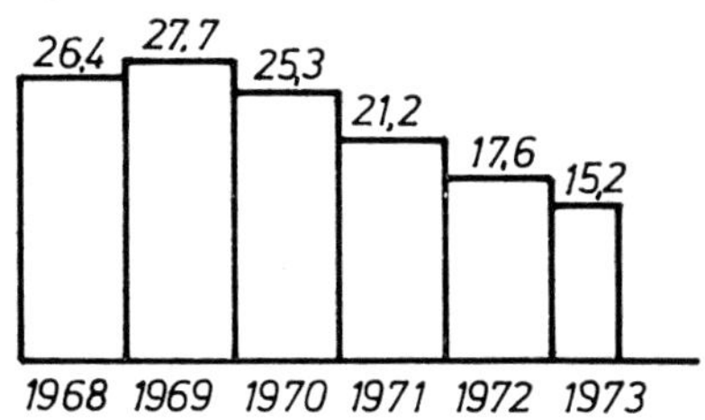

Average stay in hospital

YRS	Nº OF PATI-ENTS	EXTENSION OF BURNS															DEATHS	
		UP TO 10%			UP TO 20%			UP TO 30%			UP TO 40%			MORE THAN 50%				
		-1	-7	-14	-1	-7	-14	-1	-7	-14	-1	-7	-14	-1	-7	-14	Nº	%
1968 1973	1426	68	1016	123	7	109	20	-	34	8	1	21	2	-	14	3	18	1,2%

Fig. 1. Review of burns treated at the ward for burns of the department of Pediatric Surgery, Zagreb

made to use autografts for functionally more important areas and where there were full thickness burns. Well performed anaesthesia and an adequate accurate compensation of the blood lost make large-surface operations possible. The first dressing is performed the following day and the subsequent ones every second or third day, as required. After 8–10 days the grafts are so well fixed that physiotherapy can start. A corrective bandage is applied if necessary. The donor area epithelizes in 8 days. If homografts are used, their rejection takes place between the eighth and the fourteenth day. In dermal burns spontaneous epithelization from the preserved skin adnexa occurs in a few days. Areas where the whole skin thickness is affected develop granulations which are covered by autografts from the already epithelized donor areas. In this way we succeeded in completely autografting, in a very short time, also cases with very extensively burnt body surfaces (Fig. 1).

Conclusion

The method of early necrectomy (tangential excision) and immediate skin grafting applied in deep burns has proved successful in preventing the development of infection (which cannot be achieved by other methods) and in preserving the potentially damaged layers that would be otherwise lost. The method also prevents the development of burn disease, considerably shortens hospitalization, minimizes the formation of scars and contractures, and essentially improves the prognosis of a great many deep burns.

References

1. Jackson, D. M. (1969): Second thoughts on the burn wound. J. Trauma 9 : 839.
2. Jackson, D. M. and Stone, P. A. (1972): Tangential excision and grafting of burns. Brit. J. plast. Surg. 25 : 416.
3. Janžekovič, Z. (1970): A new concept in the early excision and immediate grafting of burns. J. Trauma 10 : 1103.
4. Janžekovič, Z. (1972): Primarna obrada velikih opekotina. Acta chir. yugosl. 19, suppl. 1.
5. Kohn, J. (1971): In: Research in Burns. H. Huber, Bern, 188.
6. Pedišić, I. (1971): Application of early necrectomy and grafting in deep dermal burns in children. In: Research in Burns. H. Huber, Bern, 295.
7. Stone, P. A. and Lawrence, J. C. (1973): Healing of tangentially excised and grafted burns in man. Brit. J. plast. Surg. 26 :.

I. P., Klaićeva 16,
41 000 Zagreb, Yugoslavia

NEW MODIFICATION OF THE MOWLEM-JACKSON METHOD

L. PASHEV and K. TROSHEV

Bulgarian Medical Academy, Medical Faculty, Varna, Bulgaria

This work presents our modification of the Mowlem-Jackson method. The essence of this modification lies in the autografts perforation of the mesh skin graft type. If the auto- and homograft ribbons are alike in width before the perforation, additional stretching of the latter increases the covering area by about 100 per cent.

Up to now we have applied this modification to six patients — children and adults — with very extensive and deep burns above 40 per cent and of third and fourth degree.

The perforation was carried out manually with a lancet of 5 to 8 mm long threads at distances of 3–5 mm. The homograft ribbons were about 2.5 cm broad. We used interrupted or continuous sutures by which nearly a double width of the autograft ribbons was obtained. The autograft taking with all our patients has been about 90–95 per cent.

In one of the patients a heavy hypoproteinaemia developed during the postoperative period, which was later overcome. Besides this a great part of the other non-perforated grafts used for covering another burn area of the patient failed to take, while the perforated ones remained and began to re-epithelize at their edges. In other patients we observed suppuration at the first dressings and presence of Pseudomonas aeruginosa, Staphylococcus aureus and Streptococcus beta-haemolyticus. Because of the good drainage of the mesh skin graft, the results were nevertheless successful. The perforated openings epithelized for about 10–12 days. Epithelization from the edges of the autografts appeared for about 30–40 days. The covered area did not differ from that of the original method of Mowlem-Jackson. We had slight or no hypertrophic reaction of the perforated openings in our patients. The extension we obtained in the different patients runs between 250–300 per cent, the difference being caused by the unequal manual perforation and by not entirely equal homograft ribbons.

Although we observed only six patients, we consider this modification to be of advantage especially at extensive burns with only small areas suitable for donor sites. It combines the advantages of the Mowlem-Jackson method, i. e. the use of homoplastic material, lenghtening of the edges after epithelisation, better aesthetical and functional results, with the advantages of the mesh skin graft: extension of the graft by about 100 per cent, good drainage, good take even under bad local circumstances and the serious condition of these patients.

L. P., ul. Shipka 26,
Varna, Bulgaria

COLLAGEN FOAMS AS A BIOLOGICAL BURN DRESSING

M. JEŽEK and K. LEIKEP

Burns Unit, Regional Hospital Ostrava, Czechoslovakia

The application of various biological materials in covering large surface wounds was described in the past in a number of papers. If this covering is to be used as a dressing, it must:

- well absorb the wound secretion,
- protect the wound from further damage,
- prevent secondary bacterial contamination,
- not damage the tissue.

The collagen foam prepared by the Research Institute for Antibiotics and Biotransformations proved to us, after many experiments with other materials, to be superior to them and to fulfill the above requirements more or less totally. Special "platelets" 4–6 mm thick, covering 8 × 10 cm were available to us. The foam is sterilized by irradiation and stored at room temperature. The application is quite simple, it is applied to the wound either dry or made wet by any aqueous solution. It can be well adapted to the wound surface and does not cause any irritation to the wound and neighbouring tissues. The speed of its solubility, enzymatic degradation, is dependent on the degree of hardening. The soft foam is dissolved at the latest in 2 days, the hardened one in 5–8 days, according to the degree of hardening. It is a very good carrier of medicaments which can be added in the process of production or immediately before its application. The antigenicity when applied topically is very low and it declines parallelly to the degree of hardening. The doses of antigen, entering the organism during its dissolution, are below the threshold levels and for this reason no immunological reaction develops. It can be assumed that collagen can act as a stimulator of fibrilogenesis as well, as proved experimentally by Weidmann and Wood. A certain part of collagen dissolved in neutral salts solutions acts as a nucleation centre in the course of the development of the fibrilar structure, thus creating "ways" where the fibroblasts move and along which new capillaries are formed. Collagen foam has the property of binding the wound secretion. In the first phase the secretion is soaked into the foam, after its dissolution a gel-like film is formed on the wound surface which effectively limits further secretions. When the film becomes dry, a subtile eschar remains, under which the wound can be healed undisturbed.

In our study, we used collagen foam in the following indications:

1. 2nd degree burns,
2. donor sites,
3. granulating surfaces after deep burns,
4. trophic remaining defects.

After careful debridement of the second-degree burn, we applied the collagen foam either dry, or made wet by saline, 3 per cent boric acid or the solution of an appropriate antibiotic. The healing proceeded smoothly; when increased secretion was observed, we applied the foam again.

The donor sites are superficial surface wounds with capillary bleeding of various intensity. Besides the dressing function, dry or wet collagen foam had in this indication a marked haemostatic effect, with subsequent speedy healing.

In deep burns, where an adequate supply of skin grafts was not available, we covered the rest of the granulating surfaces with the collagen foam, usually wet with the antibiotic chosen according to the sensitivity findings. As a result, the secretion from the granulating surfaces diminished, the accompanying activity of infection was decreased, and the general condition improved. Collagen foam was applied to granulating surfaces even as a preparatory procedure before transplantation. We noticed a good cleaning effect and revitalization of granulation as well as better taking of grafts.

The remaining trophic defects are usually the sequelae of a chronic infection or of a secondary breakdown of the healed surfaces on exposed localisations. After an abrasion of the wound bottom, dry collagen foam was applied to create a clean eschar which would not prevent the healing and to provide a temporary mechanical protection. Smaller surfaces healed spontaneously, larger ones were capable, after being cleaned, for transplantation, with a better chance of success.

Collagen foam was applied mostly as the inner part of a compressive dressing. In appropriate cases (localisations) it was used independently, without any further dressing.

We can summarize that collagen foam is very useful for local tratment of burns. Due to its advantageous storage properties and the simple application techniques, it can be available in sufficient quantities not only in specialized centers, but in all departments dealing with burns as well.

M. J., Burns Unit, Regional Hospital, Syllabova 19,
703 86 Ostrava 3, Czechoslovakia

ANAESTHESIOLOGY, RESUSCITATION AND INTENSIVE CARE

PRINCIPLES OF BURN RESUSCITATION

J. POČTA and R. KÖNIGOVÁ

Department of Anaesthesiology and Resuscitation, and Burns Centre, University Hospital, Prague, Czechoslovakia

Burn shock is a form of wound shock because of the tissue injury, but it differs from it in many respects. In addition to the extensive loss of plasma lasting 48 hours, there is also a deficiency of whole blood (by haemolysis) and of water and electrolytes. Burn shock may be complicated by thermal damage to the lung if hot gases have been inhaled.

In playing his role in treating any traumatic or surgical shock, the anaesthetist is concerned, particularly, in burn resuscitation. He assists in fluid replacement and thus in providing adequate perfusion of organs and tissues of vital importance. He aims at eliminating the causes of respiratory embarrassment and at thus preventing ventilatory insufficiency. He chooses the best method for administration of oxygen and uses all his skill and experience to relieve pain.

The principle tasks of burn resuscitation are:

I. 1. replacement of lost fluids;
   2. restoration of the blood flow in small vessels;
   3. control of the acid-base balance;

II. 1. care of open and clear upper airways:
   2. improvement of hypoxia of the whole organism by oxygen therapy;

III. relief of pain and sedation of excitation;

IV. 1. control of blood chemistry (natrium, potassium chloride, urea, creatinine);
   2. parenteral feeding, i.e. adequate supply of proteins, calories, vitamins;
   3. to contribute to design the burn "formula diet".

Initial estimation of the amount of fluids during the 48 hours from the time of burning is made on the basis of various formulae (Evans, Brook, Moore). All of them help as schemes, which have to be modified according to the previous treatment before admission and according to the patient's response. We must also consider the stress and strain before and immediately after injury and the delay in the initiation of treatment. We put emphasis on adequate and early anti-shock therapy, i.e. the balance between the sufficient intravascular volume and the increase of oedema; an early ansti-hock therapy means to start the fluid replacement not later than after four hours. Secondly, we fight against vasoconstriction which is pronounced, particularly, in severe burns. This is why we do not see the classical signs of shock such as fall of blood pressure but tachycardia, too, appears later than might be expected. The reliable control is in urine output. To prevent fatal consequences of vasoconstriction, we try to eliminate it by applying dehydrobenzperidol (single dose 1 ml = 2.5 mg per 10 kg of weight) after four to six hours. We are aware of the fact that by opening the peripheral blood vessels we may increase the metabolic acidosis because of products of anaerobic metabolism. For correction we use a 5 per cent solution of natrium bicarbonate.

The anaesthetist participates in the prevention of respiratory embarrassment together with the ENT specialist. Laryngospasm or bronchospasm following exposure to toxic vapours or smoke require bronchodilator drugs. Laryngeal oedema develops in face and neck burns when the accident occurs in a closed space. It is usually transitory and may be overcome by endotracheal intubation. Hot gases and steam irritate the tracheo-bronchial tree and excessive secretion obstructs the airways, which may result in pulmonary oedema caused by high intrapulmonary pressure. This condition indicates tracheotomy for performing continuous toilet of the airways.

All severe burns (i.e. over 20 per cent of body surface) are treated permanently with oxygen, administered by means of a nasopharyngeal catheter.

We lay stress upon relief of pain for two reasons: first, to limit the production of catecholamines as a part of anti-shock treatment, secondly, to calm the excitation of the patient and to prevent psychiatric disturbances.

The shifts of minerals are often related to shifts in the acido-base balance. The correction is part of the overall treatment. From the second week we find hypopotassaemia together with respiratory alkalosis responding to potassium chloride.

In parenteral feeding, dried plasma is indispensable apart from albumin — in adults and native plasma in children in the treatment of septicemia. When solutions of amino-acids are available we use them together with concentrated solutions of carbohydrates. Our scheme of realimentation provides the patient with 3000 calories in 24 hours. Peroral diet is indicated as soon as the patient is able to eat. During the first 48–72 hours we offer alternately a spoonful of tea and milk to prevent shock — induced mucosal lesions in the stomach and duodenum. Later, the peroral diet is dependent upon gastrointestinal, liver, kidney and other complications. The necessity of applying general anaesthesia every second day or even daily interferes with the need for regular peroral intake. We endeavour to solve this problem by giving the severely burned a so-called "protein breakfast", between 5 and 6 a.m. to prevent then from starving 15 hours or even more.

All severe burns require immediate intensive care just as any severe injury, but it must not be discontinued after the shock period has been overcome. On the contrary, the patient subsequently requires not only intensive care, but it becomes extensive in view of the multiple aspects from which the patient must be treated during the whole period of burn illness. Better results might be achieved if a team of specialists is ready to be consulted and if there is closest cooperation, at any time, between the surgeon and the anaesthetist.

J. P., Tř. Obránců míru 107,
160 00 Praha 6, Czechoslovakia

ANAESTHESIA FOR EARLY EXCISION OF EXTENSIVE FULL-THICKNESS BURNS

R. E. SPIJKER

The Red Cross Hospital, Beverwijk, The Netherlands

For full-thickness burns early excision is more and more often becoming the treatment of choice. Serious undernourishment and bacterial invasion can be kept within limits while often shorter healing times and better functions are gained. The best moment for excision lies within the first four postburn days.

The excised areas can be covered with skin grafts. When there is not enough donor site available spreading techniques such as the Meek-Wall procedure or the meshgrafts are used. Because the results are satisfactory there is a tendency to increase the percentage of body surface area that is excised.

Because of the considerations mentioned above the anaesthetist is confronted with some problems. Yet it appears in practice that these patients bear anaesthesia better than in a later phase when they are debilitated and septic, on the understanding that some precautions are taken.

The most important of these is the control of the water, electrolyte and blood balance. Before anaesthesia it must be ensured shock is well treated, circulating volume and cardiac output are normal, urine production is sufficient and there is no acidosis.

During the operation blood loss should be minimised as much as possible and the blood which is lost has to be replaced fully.

Burned patients lose much water through evaporation from the burned surface. After excision this evaporation is maximal. The lost water has to be replaced. The heat energy which is used for the evaporation is at normal surrounding temperatures withdrawn from the patient. So he loses more heat than normal and he may develop a strong tendency to shiver. During the operation care should be taken that the patient cools down as little as possible.

Metabolism goes up. Oxygen consumption and carbon dioxide delivery are increased. Ventilation is also increased. In many patients gas-diffusion in the lungs is disturbed and there may be shunting. This results in a lowered oxygensaturation often combined with a lowered carbondioxide-concentration.

During anaesthesia supervision of ventilation and oxygenation is necessary.

Some practical considerations: The operating theatre should be warm. 25–30 degrees of centigrade is a desirable temperature. Relative humidity may be low. Cool airstreams must be prevented.

To keep the operation as short as possible the operating teams should consist of several surgeons. Some of them can perform the excision while others take off split skin and prepare meshgrafts.

In order to limit blood loss in excision of extremities they should be supported in a vertical position. We prefer this over the tourniquet-method because after taking off the tourniquet bleeding may occur causing haematomas under the grafts. The necrotic skin is not meticulously cut off but we use more pulling than cutting because in this way it is easier to find natural cleavage and there is less bleeding. So far we have not been obliged to use hypotension. The amount of blood lost is estimated and replaced during the operation. We give fresh blood — 1 to 7 days old — because it has best conserved oxygen carrying capacity. Circulation is supervised by means of measuring arterial and central venous pressure, capnography and urine production.

If the amount of haemoglobine goes down in the following days more blood is given until a haemoglobine of at least 8mMol/L is reached.

In a group of our patients an average of 100 ml of blood is needed for every percent of excised body surface area.

In regard to the need for water and electrolytes we use the rule of Brooke hospital for the not excised burned surface area. The evaporational water loss from the excised area may be 50–200 ml of water per one per cent excision which is substituted as a glucose solution. An increase of serum sodium often means water shortage.

What demand do we make on anaesthesia? Sufficient analgesia should be provided for. The anaesthetic should not increase the tendency to produce shock caused by hypovolaemia. A high percentage of oxygen — 40 per cent — in the inspired gases is needed. The ventilation must be sufficient for the increased metabolism. All patients are intubated without the use of succinylcholine because of the possibility of cardiac arrest. When intubation is not possible because there is edema of head and neck, the operation should be postponed for one day.

We have evaluated three methods of anaesthesia:

1. Pentothal, intubation after giving nondepolarising relaxants e.g. Pavulon. Controlled ventilation with gas and oxygen in a ratio of 6 to 4 and high dosis of narcotisc e.g. Nicomorfine or neuroleptanalgesia. The ventilation has to be monitored by capnography (end tidal carbon dioxide measuring) as often as from 50 to 100 per cent elevated ventilation volume is required. Remarkable is that patients have little shivering after operation.
2. Induction with gas and halothane, intubation without relaxation and then procede to penthrane. We have the patient breathing spontaneously with periodic hyperinflation. This method is less satisfying when the operation lasts longer than two hours.
3. Ketalar we only used for small excisions of patients with facial burns. For children it is a satisfying method. A disadvantage is the period of fearfull dreams after the operation in patients who are already psycholabile.

During anaesthesia we check:

1. Arterial pressure with Riva-Rocci or in combination with a pulse monitor.
2. Central venous pressure. This is especially important to prevent overfilling in patients with small circulatory reserves.
3. Capnography. This is a monitoring of the carbon dioxide in the expiratory gases. It gives information of ventilation but can also give information of the circulation.
4. Urine production. Oliguria with a good arterial pressure is an indication of hypovolaemia.

5. Pulse rate. The value of it is difficult to judge as it is influenced by many causes.
6. Electrocardiography.

Contraindications against early excision are in our opinion only serious burning of the lungs and serious renal failure. Till now we have not yet performed excisions of more than 40 per cent full thickness burned body surface area. A bad condition of the patient caused by a preexisting heart-lung disease and neurological diseases produces to our experience very increased risks but we feel the chance of survival with conservative treatment should be at least as bad.

Summarising it can be stated that early excision of extensive full-thickness burns is a promising method of treatment and does not necessarily produce unsurmountable difficulties for the anaesthesia and resuscitation of the patient.

R. E. S., Dreef 31, Beverwijk, The Netherlands

ANAESTHESIA AND RESUSCITATION IN BURNED CHILDREN

L. KOPECKÁ and M. DRAPKA

Department of Anaesthesiology and Resuscitation of the Faculty Hospital in Prague-Motol, Czechoslovakia

Burns are injuries causing a serious general disease, when affecting a larger surface of the body. Unlike adults, small children are more endangered, because of their considerable anatomical, physiological and psychological peculiarities. Children have a thin skin, the relation of the body surface to the body weight is far higher than in adults. The tracheal diameter is small, the glomerulotubular function is not developed, and the peripheral circulation is unstable. A burned child does not easily tolerate the changes in the body-fluid balance, the temperature of the surrounding medium and psychological influences. Children are much more inclined to vomit and to have cramps. A critically burned suckling has no self-preservation instinct, and the therapy has therefore to be more exact, to keep the child in most stabilized conditions.

In the years 1971–1972, 80 children up to three years of age were treated in the Department for Pediatric Surgery of the Faculty Hospital in Prague-Motol with burns on 20 to 80 per cent of body surface. The cooperation of the anaesthetist was usually requested immediately after admission of the burned patient, not only because of necessary anaesthesia during surgical treatment, but first of all to start with the therapy of the shock condition which is always present in more serious burns. We helped when vitally important functions — mainly the cardiorespiratory apparatus — failed, further to improve the inner medium and to supress pain. Extensively burned children or burns of especially algic body regions require a complex therapy in the struggle against often destructive pain. According to literature, psychical changes occur in 80 per cent of children with burns affecting more than 10 per cent of their body surface. Each handling such an injured child is a source of algic and shock symptoms usually further deteriorating its serious condition. Analgesy and sedation is of especial importance in such cases. This is why we immediately in the earliest stage administer the neuroplegical mixtures M_1, M_k, and if necessary M_2, too. We give the mixture in the condition of shock and in excessive excitation intravenously, later intramuscularly. The medium dose is 1 ml per 8 kg of body weight per day. When cramps occur, we add valium, intravenously or intramuscularly, according to the seriousness of the disease.

In surgical treatment of a burned patient we try to minimize the physical and psychical traumatisation. For a child, general anaesthesia is incontestably the most effective and psychically least burdening method. We made good experience with the use of Ketamine chloride, whose powerful analgetic effect and maintenance of vegetative stability substituted the inhalatory form of anaesthesia. We give it intravenously in doses of 1–2 mg per kg of body weight, or 6–8 mg per kg of body weight intramuscularly. The intramuscular application is of advantage in small children, especially when access to the veins is difficult because of the burns. In the Ketalar anaesthesia, it is not necessary to use the mask, which is difficult in burns of the face, where the mask is not only a source of infection but also makes it impossible to properly treat these regions. The patient in Ketalar anaesthesia is not connected with the narcosis apparatus and can be handled freely as required for the surgical treatment. This is made possible by Ketalar itself by its stabilizing the vegetative functions; there consequently do not occur dangerous deteriorations in the patient's condition caused by position changes, as in the case of other anaesthetics. We abandoned the strong premedications, regularly applied in other operations, and give only atropine, because of the early awaking of the patients and to ensure their necessary intake of food. For the same reason, we let children starve for the shortest possible time before anaesthesia, that means for about 4 hours. Not even during repeated application of Ketalar — in one case ten times in two weeks as it is necessary in dressing, bathing, surgical treatment — did we observe adverse effects.

In patients in a serious shock condition, when the basic vital functions fail, and when oxidation of the tissues is insufficient — which we assess not only according to clinical observation, but in the first place according to a control of the blood gases according to Astrup — we insert an endotracheal tube, in order to ensure sufficient oxygen supply and, if necessary, auxiliary or controlled breathing. If we need relaxation for the intubation or for controlled breathing, we avoid the application of succinylcholine because of its vagotonic effect on the heart. This risk is especially high in burned patients who show a high incidence of hyperpotassaemia.

In case of high temperature caused by sepsis, we do not hesitate to induce hypothermy.

General anaesthesia in reparative plastic operations in burns does not differ from routine anaesthesia.

References

1. Doleček, R. and Kalina, J. (1970): Léčení popálených. Avicenum, Praha.
2. Jadrný, J. (1960): Úskalí anestesie při komplikujících onemocněních. SZdN, Praha.
3. Matter, P. (1971): In: Research in Burns. H. Huber, Bern.
4. Počta, J. (1972): The choise of anaesthesia in burned. (P. 264) Advances in Anaesthesiology and Resuscitation. Avicenum, Praha.
5. Smith, R. M. (1959): Anesthesia for Infants and Children. The C. V. Mosby Company, St. Louis.

L. K., Kukučinova 1147,
142 00 Praha 4, Czechoslovakia

ANALGESIA IN THE TREATMENT OF BURNS

E. JÍCHOVÁ, D. KŘUPKOVÁ and J. POČTA

Department of Anaesthesiology and Resuscitation, University Hospital, Prague, Czechoslovakia

The importance of analgesic methods in modern anaesthesiology is growing. We require analgetics to have the following properties:

1. relatively low toxicity,
2. suitability for all age groups,
3. wide indication possibilities in severe, complicated cases,
4. prompt effect,
5. negligible side effects,
6. no effect on breathing and blood circulation,
7. multivarious application forms (injection solutions, capsules, tablets, drops, solutions for local application, etc.),
8. low cost,
9. preference is given to analgetics which are not subject to opium law restrictions.

At present, there seems to be no doubt that performance of analgesia should be the domain of anaesthetists. Anaesthetists indicate and prescribe analgetics in the following situations:

a) post-operative pain,
b) pain connected with tumorous growths,
c) post-traumatic pain,
d) painful dressing of burn wounds, painful baths of burned patients, etc.

In the treatment of burns, analgetic methods are indispensable during primary debridement, in changing dressing and in other minor surgical procedures (including baths). All these procedures are highly painful, must be repeated several times a week and may have a very enervating effect on the patient.

At present, the following methods may be considered:

a) neuroleptanalgesia in repeated low doses (2–3 ml in adults),
b) dissociative anaesthesia by Ketamine in 0.5–1 mg/kg body weight, applied i.v.,
c) methoxyflurane analgesia (0.3–0.4 per cent concentration),
d) highly effective analgetics: 1. pentazocine - Fortral,
   2. piritramide — Dipidolor,
   3. tilidine — Valoron,

e) electroanalgesia, electrohypnosis,
f) combination of classical analgetics such as: diazepam + promethazin + pethidin,
g) local anaesthesia.

a) Neuroleptanalgesia covers wide indication possibilities and should be preferred to neuroplegics for the following reasons:
   - lower toxicity for parenchymatous organs,
   - low frequency of side-effects,
   - shorter period of drowsiness,
   - analgesic effect is higher, while vital functions (breathing, circulation) are not affected as much as with neuroplegics,
   - the return of full consciousness is more prompt.
b) Dissociative anaesthesia by Ketamine is preferred by many specialists; in combination with dehydrobenzperidole premedication, complications are becoming very rare. Very low doses must be prescribed individually according to the age, weight and general condition of the patient (1 mg i.v.).
c) Methoxyflurane analgesia is being successfully used in many institutions. In this country it is unfortunately applied very rarely for lack of necessary technical equipment.
d) Highly effective analgetics, such as pentazocine, piritramide, tilidine are being used in our department quite frequently and with good results. However, they should not be applied in combination with other analgetics and opiates to avoid complications.

The characteristic properties of these three potent analgetics are compared in Table 1.

TABLE 1.

Comparison of characteristics of three potent analgetics — pentazocine, tilidine and piritramide

	Pentazocine	Tilidine	Piritramide
Toxicity	0	0	0
Age groups	all	all	all
Indication range	wide	wide	wide
Onset after	30 mins	15 mins	20 mins
Side effects	nausea	minimal	practically none
Influence on breathing and circulation	0	0	0
Aplication forms	i.v., i.m., p.o.	i.v., i.m., p.o., p.r.	i.v., i.m.
Opiate law	0	0	+
Addiction	0	0	+

e) Electroanalgesia, electrohypnosis — from the toxicity aspect, these methods should be the safest. So far, however, small advance has been achieved in our country for lack of necessary technical co-operation. Experimental results obtained so far are highly satisfactory and convincing. These may be the methods of the future.
f) Combination of some classical analgetics, such as diazepam and promethazin and pethidin, or combination of diazepam with minute doses of Pentothal have yielded satisfactory results. We used the above analgetics combination in a limited number of cases with good results in the following doses: diazepam 10 mg, promethazin and pethidin 50 mg, Pentothal about 200 mg i.v. The effect lasted up to 30 mins.
g) The indication of local anaesthesia in the treatment of burns is limited, but should be

considered in individual cases. It may be applied for surgical procedures on the upper extremities (brachial plexus blockade, axillar blockade).

We presented a brief evaluation of modern analgetic methods which may be recommended for the treatment of burns. We hope that in the future new possibilities of analgesia of burns will emerge with the development of electroanaesthesia.

E. J., Faculty Hospital, Dept. of Anaesthesiology,
Šrobárova 50,
100 34 Praha 10, Czechoslovakia

KETALAR IN PREMEDICATION OF CHILDREN

T. SOTORNÍKOVÁ and J. SKÁCEL

Regional Hospital, Department of Anaesthesiology and Resuscitation, Ostrava, Czechoslovakia

The purpose of premedication is the following:
to tranquillize the patient, to reduce undesirable reflexes by means of vagolytic action, to supress excessive salivation and to prevent vomiting as well as to secure atraumatic introduction into general anaesthesia and to diminish the whole consumption of anaesthetic agents.

Up to the present time we did not have an ideal drug which would fulfil all requirements in this way and the desirable actions could be reached only by a combination of various medicaments.

The introduction into general anaesthesia in children is usually realised by means of inhaling anaesthesia. This is very often complicated by the fear and the crying of children. Potentiated premedication which is used at many anaesthesiological departments has its advantages as well as undesirable complications.

At our department, we used various combinations of drugs in the premedication of children. But we had no drug without risk which could be applied at the department and which could provide a premedication effect and simultaneously facilitate the introduction into general anaesthesia. A new drug, Ketalar, is a medicament which can fulfil all these requirements. It can be applied intramuscularly and when the dose applied in this way is less than 5 mg per 1 kg of body weight, no side effects are visible in the cardio-pulmonary system and both unconsciousness and analgesia are achieved with a retention of laryngeal and pharyngeal reflexes. Ketalar can be applied together with atropine and it can be combined with all anaesthetic agents. These are further advantages of this drug.

Methods

We used Ketalar in 105 children in the premedication. Their age was ranging from 4 months to 14 years. The doses which we used were 2 mg/kg in 62 children, 2.5 mg/kg in 32 children and 3 mg/kg in 10 children. Ketalar was applied together with atropine intramuscularly. The atropine dose was 0.1 mg/5 kg. This kind of premedication was applied from 10 to 20 min. before starting general anaesthesia. The children fell asleep gradually within 5 min. after they had been given the premedication. After being asleep they were transferred to the operating theatre. Both the introduction and the maintenance of general anaesthesia were provided by a mixture of Narcotan, N_2O and O_2. In children, who got this kind of premedication, the blood-pressure and the pulse-rate were measured 5 min. after the premedication, during anaesthesia, and after the operation had been finished. We simultaneously observed side effects such as nausea and vomiting, clonus-twitches and hallucinations. We found that within 5 min. after application of Ketalar together with atropine the blood-pressure increased in 55 per cent of our patients by an average of about 20 mmHg, in 20 per cent fell by about 15 mmHg on an average, and in 25 per cent it remained unchanged. The pulse-rate rose in all patients by about 10 to 25 per cent. The blood-pressure fell during general anaesthesia in 60 per cent out of all anaesthetised patients by about 15 mmHg in comparison with preanaesthetic levels. In 15 per cent of anaesthetised patients the blood-pressure increased by about 10 mmHg. The pulse-rate did not change during general anaesthesia in comparison with findings after premedication. When the operation was finished the blood-pressure remained elevated in 30 per cent by about 10 mmHg and fell in 35 per cent by about 10 mmHg; the pulse-rate was in 70 per cent the same as before premedication and in 30 per cent there persisted mild tachycardia.

As regards side-effects we observed in 5 p.c. nausea and vomiting, in 6 p.c. purposeless movements, in 2 p.c. hallucinations and one child got clonus-twitches. The children were allocutionable and had unaltered reflexes immediately after the operation was finished. Postoperative analgesia lasted 2.5 to 3 hours. We did not observe any depression of breathing.

Discussion

The onset of the stage of tolerance after i.m. application of Ketalar comes by degrees within 3 to 4 min. The patient loses contact with his enviroment and with his own body. This stage was reached after Ketalar application at doses from 2.5 to 3 mg, which is in agreement with the statements by Erdmann and Fray, When a dose of 2 mg was used, the stage of tolerance was reached only in 45 per cent. The time factor is of the same importance as the dose of Ketalar. The most advantageous time for the start of general anaesthesia is in an interval between 10 and 15 min. after the application of Ketalar. The stage of tolerance mostly disappears after 20 min.

Ketalar has a stimulating effect on the cardiovascular system in contrast to other anaesthetic agents. This was expressed by an acceleration of the pulse-rate in all children and by an elevation of blood-pressure in 55 per cent of children. The changes in blood-pressure and in the pulse-rate over general anaesthesia were caused by Narcotan and other factors.

Side effects, which are described in Ketalar anaesthesia, are very rare when Ketalar is used in this way.

The children were allocutionable and had unaltered reflexes after the operation had been finished. Analgesia and somnolence were lasting from 2.5 to 3 hours and after 3 hours children were able to eat and did not vomit.

Conclusions

Ketalar as a premedication drug has the following advantages:

1. It can be applied together with atropine intramuscularly and can be used in combination with other anaesthetic agents.
2. This kind of premedication makes possible quiet introduction into general anaesthesia.

3. The child is transferred sleeping to the operating theatre and is in this way spared undesirable psychic traumatisation.
4. After the end of general anaesthesia, there follows a quick return of the reflexes.
5. Analgesia and somnolence with retention of the reflexes are lasting from 2.5 to 3 hours after the end of general anaesthesia.
6. In the burns centres, the children are nursed many times in general anaesthesia over one hospitalisation. This is why their premedication with Ketalar is highly advantageous, apart from possibilities to continue in general anaesthesia only by means of the mixture of N_2O and O_2, which is quite adequate for small surgical operations in burned patients.

T. S., Dukelská 3,
750 00 Přerov, Czechoslovakia

GENERAL ANAESTHESIA IN EXPERIMENTAL BURN SHOCK IN PIGLETS

M. VOJNOV

General Hospital, Maribor, Yugoslavia

To investigate the cause of the burn shock, we decided to use as the main means of anaesthesia Ketalar (Ketamin hydrochloride) on Landrace piglets.

Thirty minutes before the anaesthesia 22 piglets, aged 6–11 weeks, were administered intramuscularly 1 mg of atropine and 10–15 mg of Valium (Diazepam).

After the first intramuscular dose of Ketalar (20 mg/kg body weight), the piglet was anaesthetised after 3–4 minutes. The additional intravenous application of Thalamonal (1.5 ml/10 kg body weight) and local 1 p.c. Xylocain spray in rima glotidis made it possible to intubate the animals orotracheally without relaxation. They were connected to an anaesthesia apparatus of the Dräger-type-circular system. The animals were breathing the mixture of $O_2 : N_2O$ in proportion of 50 : 50 per cent, partly spontaneously and partly controlled.

Further additional doses of Ketalar were — if necessary — administered intravenously (15 mg/kg body weight), the same as the doses of Dehydrobenzperidol or Fentanyl.

The piglets were completely quiet after being submerged for 30 seconds into 80 degrees of centigrade water resulting in 5–50 per cent burns of total body surface; however, we had the impression that with the raised temperature the dose of anaesthetics had to be increased.

The anaesthesia was effective during the whole experimental operation, from the intubation and the connection of temperature and other measuring sounds, and during the observation of the course of the burn shock, which could last for five or more hours. The course and the depth of the anaesthesia was adequate in the described experiment.

The temperature was registered with temperatures measuring sounds in various parts of the body with the help of Elema — Schönander apparatus.

The ECG apparatus was permanently connected and periodically registered.

The blood pressure was measured in the femoral artery. The central venous pressure was measured by means of the Pfrimmer system. The blood samples for gas analysis were taken several times during the investigation. The blood picture, hematocrit, electrolytes in serum, and enzymes were determined before and after burn. The blood volume was measured by the Evans — blue method.

* Research work No. 334 045 2/12-1971, supported by Boris Kidrič Fund, Ljubljana.

RESULTS

During the described anaesthesia with Ketalar plus Thalamonal plus O_2 and N_2O, fairly stable blood circulation was observed at the beginning of anaesthesia and was not affected by severe burn shock, evident by heavy acidosis in 40–50 p.c. burns in spite of breathig the mixture of $O_2 : N_2O$ in 50 : 50 p.c. proportion.

REFERENCES

1. CORSSEN, G. and DOMINO, E. F. (1960): Dissociative anaesthesia: Further pharmacological studies and first clinical experience with the phencyclidine derivative Cl-581, Anaesth. Analg. 45 : 29.
2. GERSMEYER, E. F. und YASARGIL, E. C. (1970): Schock und Kolaps-Fibel. Stuttgart.
3. GJESSINF, J. (1968): Ketamine (Cl-581) in clinical anaesthesia. Acta anaesthes. scand. 12 : 15.
4. KING, C. H. and STEPHAN, C. R. (1967): A new intravenous or intramuscular anaestetic. Anaesthesiology 28 : 258.
5. KREUSCHNER, H. and GROTE, J. (1967): Effect of the phencyclidine derivative ketamine (Cl-581) on brain circulation and oxygen utilization in dogs. Anaesthesist 16 : 304.
6. ROBERTS, F. W. and THOMPSON, W. F. (1968): Neuroleptanalgesia in the management of mass burn cases. Med. J. Australia 1 : 128.
7. WYLIE, W. D. (1970): A Practice of Anaesthesia, Lloyd-Luke, London.

M. V., General Hospital,
Dept. of Anaesthesiology,
6200 Maribor, Yugoslavia

INFUSION THERAPY OF BURNS WITH DEXTRAN AND RINGER LACTATE 2 1/2 YEARS' RESULTS OF A CONTROLLED TRIAL

K. V. HALL and B. SØRENSEN

Department of Plastic Surgery and the Burns Unit, Kommunehospitalet, University of Copenhagen, Denmark

Introduction

Should colloids or pure electrolytes be preferred in the treatment of burn shock? This remains still an unsolved question. In the Burns Unit in Copenhagen plasma was used over a two year period (5), physiological saline over another two year period (6), and for the last six years colloid infusion, Dextran, has been used (7). The experience gained gave no indication as to which of these three methods was the best.

Material

In an attempt to derive positive information, we began a random controlled trial on 1. 2. 1971. Patients were treated either by Ringer Lactate infusion as described by Baxter (1), or by Dextran, as described by Evans from Roehampton (3). The results from the first year of the study appear in the next Issue of the Scandinavian Journal of Plastic and Reconstructive Surgery (4). This paper gives the results of the first 2 ½ years, a total of 90 patients.

Results

Patients were randomly selected after age, and extent and cause of burn (Table 1.). Forty-seven received Dextran infusions, and 43, Ringer Lactate. Estimated area of burn (E.A.B.) was greater than 40 per cent in 22 patients. Eleven patients were above 60 years of age.

Table 2 records the parameters in each of the patient groups as totals for each group (above), and as averages (below).

Despite the randomization, the groups differ, as the Ringer treated group comprises more patients with very extensive burns than the Dextran group.

There was no significant difference in the mortality in the two groups — neither as

---

* Supported by a grant from Statens Laegevidenskabelige Forskningsfond and Kong Christian den X's Fond.

TABLE 1

Cause of Burns

	Scalding	Flame	Contact	Total
Dextran	10	35	2	47
Ringer	10	31	2	43

TABLE 2

Severity of injury in the Series

Total series	No. of patients	Total body weight kg	Expected mortality (Bull a. Fischer)	Actual mortality	Area of burning sq m
Dextran	47	2244	14.9	9	19.5
Ringer	43	2503	17.1	8	24.4

Average per patient	No. of patients	Average body weight kg	Average expected mortality (Bull a. Fischer)	Area of burning s.q.m.	Average E.A.B. per cent
Dextran	47	47.7	0.3	0.41	30
Ringer	43	58.2	0.4	0.57	35

TABLE 3

Intake of Sodium and Fluid (adults only)

Adults only	0–24 hrs post burn		0–48 hrs post burn	
	sodium mEq/kg BW	fluid per cent BW	sodium mEq/kg BW	fluid per cent BW
Dextran (26)	7.84	12.2	11.58	21.8
Ringer (31)	19.86	17.9	20.88	27.7

TABLE 4

Calculated fluid volume and fluid volume actually given. Volumes expressed as percentages of initial body Weight. (Adults only)

	0–24 hrs		24–48 hrs		0–48 hrs	
	calculated	given	calculated	given	calculated	given
Dextran (26)	9.1	12.1	6.4	9.6	15.5	21.8
Ringer (31)	14.5	17.9	10	9.8	24.5	28.7

calculated from the numbers in each group, nor by comparison with the predicted mortality according to Bull and Fischer (2). Evaluation from this parameter thus does not demonstrate any difference between the two methods.

Table 3 shows the fluid volume and quantity of sodium given over the first 24 hours, and the first 48 hours, respectively. In simplification, only adult patients are included in the table, 57 in all. It is apparent that the patients in the Ringer group received 50 percent more fluid, and nearly three times as much sodium as the patients in the Dextran group within the first 24 hours. By contrast, in the second 24 hour period the Ringer group patients received virtually no sodium. The two treatment methods are, thus, basically different.

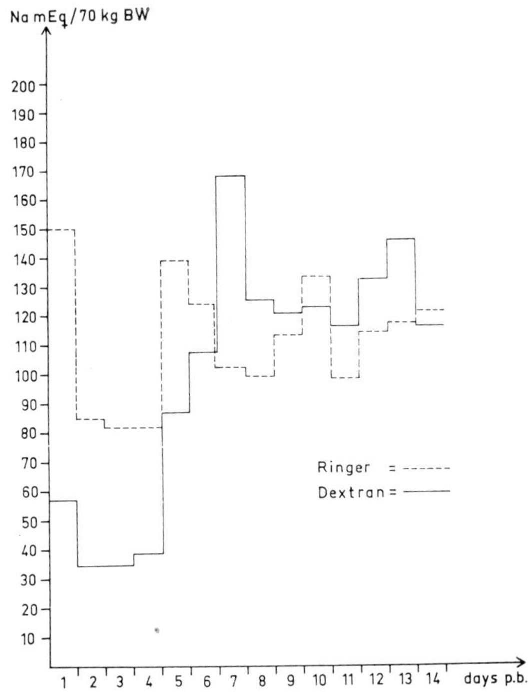

Fig. 1. Sodium output in 57 adult patients.

Table 4 shows the relationship between the fluid requirement calculated from the respective formulae, and the actual fluid volume administered. This table also concerns only adult patients. Both groups received extra fluid over the first 24 hours.

The volume given over 48 hours to the Dextran group patients requires some explanation. Table 5 summarizes the amount of fluid given over the first 48 hours in each of a series of five studies. The first two were made before the controlled trial was begun, and the volume administered was, respectively, 17.9 and 19.0 percent of initial body weight. In study 3, which will appear in Scand. J. Plast. Reconstr. Surg. (4), and which covers the first year of the controlled trial, the volume given was 25.3 percent of initial body

TABLE 5

Average fluid intake in the first 48 hours post burn in different series of patients treated by Dextran. Actual fluid intake of patients during the two first days expressed as a percentage of initial body weight.

Figures from different series treated by Dextran. (Adults only)

1. Sørensen et al.	1965:	17.9%
2. Sørensen	1971:	19.0%
3. Hall a. Sørensen	1973 a:	25.3%
4. Hall a. Sørensen	1973 b:	19.3%
5. Hall a. Sørensen	1973 c:	21.8%

TABLE 6

Hourly urine production in ml (adults only)

Adults only	No. of patients	Mean hourly urine output first 24 hrs	Mean hourly urine output second 24 hrs
Dextran	26	65	54
Ringer	31	100	102

weight. This was due to a misinterpretation of an incomplete instruction, and the correction of the instruction has entailed that the volume given over the last 18 months (study 4, Hall + Sørensen, 1973b — not to be published) is again "back to normal", at 19.3 per cent of initial body weight.

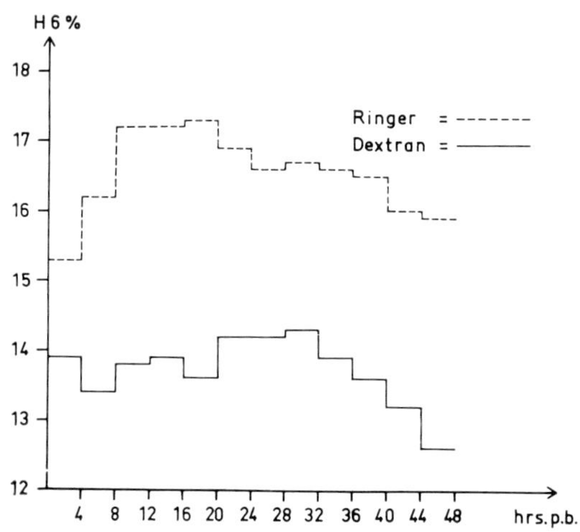

Fig. 2. Average haemoglobin values in 90 patients.

This present study consists of the series Nos. 3 and 4, and therefore the average Dextran administration seems still to be high, viz. 21.8 percent of initial body weight.

Fluid excretion is measured by taking hourly diuresis for the first 48 hours, *Table 6* shows the average results for adults. The Dextran formula is designed to give a diuresis of 60 ml/h, and actual diuresis was close to this "ideal" — 65 ml/h over the first 24 hours, and 54 ml/h over the second. In the Ringer patients, as in others treated with saline, diuresis was predictably higher.

Urinary sodium excretion was measured over the first 14 days. *Fig. 1* gives the findings in the 57 adult patients, expressed as sodium excretion in milli-equivalents in a patient of initial body weight of 70 kg. The average excretion in the average patient can thus be read directly from the curve. It is characteristic that sodium excretion in the Dextran

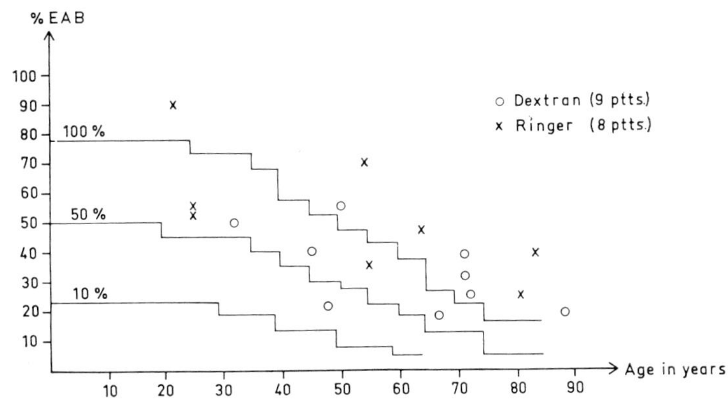

Fig. 3. Mortality

group was very low over the first days, but virtually normal in the Ringer group. This suggests that the Ringer Lactate régime in this respect may be more "physiological" than the Dextran régime.

Fig. 2 gives the average haemoglobin concentrations in all 90 patients in the first 48 hours. Haemoconcentration is more marked in the Ringer group, statistically with high significance from 8 hours onwards. If the corresponding curve for patients with E.A.B. greater than 40 per cent is constructed, similar results are obtained. Thus, in this respect Dextran would appear to be the more "physiological" treatment method.

Evaluation of results depends not only on crude mortality, which was not statistically different in the two groups, but also on the time of death, the cause of death, and the calculated mortality for the dead patients (2).

Calculated mortality is shown in *Fig. 3*, as Bull and Fischer's scheme with the 9 dead Dextran patients marked as 0, and the 8 dead Ringer patients marked as X.

Ten of the 17 patients, who died, had an expected mortality of 100 per cent, and only 1 a calculated mortality of less than 50 per cent.

Conclusions

We are still not able to give an answer to the question: colloids or pure electrolytes.

Treatment with pure electrolytes entails haemoconcentration, but a near normal sodium excretion. Dextran vice-versa.

Both treatment methods, properly clinically handled, can prevent anuria. Pulmonary oedema has not occurred.

Mortality, time and cause of death do not show statistically significant difference between the two groups.

The study is continued.

REFERENCES

1. BAXTER, C. S. T. (1968): Physiological response to crystalloid resuscitation of severe burns. Ann. N.Y. Acad. Sci. 150 : 874.
2. BULL, J. P. and FISCHER, A. J. (1954): A study of mortality in a Burns Unit; a revised estimate. Ann. Surg. 139 : 269.
3. EVANS, A. J. (1957): Experience in a Burn Unit. Brit. med. J. 50 : 547.
4. HALL, K. V. and SØRENSEN, B. (1973): The treatment of Burn Shock. A comparative controlled trial of treatment by colloid infussion (Dextran-Saline), and by exclusively electrolyte infusion (Ringer Lactate). Scand. J. plast. reconstr. Surg. 7 : 67.
5. SPRECHLER, M., BACKER, O. and BADEN, H. (1960): Centraliseret behandling af forbrændinger Ugeskr. læger 122: 815.
6. SØRENSEN, B. and SEJRSEN, P. (1965): Saline solutions in the treatment of burn shock. Acta chir. scand. 129 : 239.
7. SØRENSEN, B. (1971): Fluid therapy with Dextran. In: Contemporary Burn Management (ed. Polk, H. C. Jr., and Stone, H.). Little, Brown and Co., Boston, 71.

B. S., Toftholm Allé 12,
2900 Hellerup, Denmark

ORAL INGESTION OF AN ELECTROLYTE SOLUTION AS SHOCK PROPHYLAXIS IN BURN PATIENTS

F. W. AHNEFELD, R. H. BORST and R. BARDUA

Department of Anaesthesiology, University of Ulm, 7900 Ulm, F.R.G.

After burns a hypovolaemia occurs which is of considerable importance for the development of burn shock. The organism tries to reduce the resulting deficit in volume by intravascular influx of interstitial fluid. Therefore, the volume of the interstice is very important for this endogenous compensation.

Loss in blood volume after burns

Our investigations on 20 burn patients show that the decrease of the intravascular volume commences immediately after trauma. As table 1 shows, the average deficit in volume amounts to nearly 900 ml 30 to 60 minutes after a second degree burn of approximately 22 per cent of the body surface, that is about 18 per cent of the blood volume. After a further 3 hours, the loss climbs to about 30 per cent of the blood volume. The same is valid for electrical burns. The consequences of a hypovolaemia for the circulation and tissue perfusion are evident: a rise in the diastolic blood pressure, a tachycardia as well as an uncompensated metabolic acidosis result.

TABLE 1.

Results of investigations on burn patients: a) burns by flames, steam and other sources; scalding, b) electrical burn patients

	Time after burning (min)	Per cent of burn area	Deficit of volume ml	per cent	Blood pressure (mm Hg)	Pulse rate	$pH_{art.}$	$pCO_{2art.}$ (mm Hg)
	30–60	22.4	894	18.3	128/ 90	96	7.394	38
a	60–120	27.3	1268	24.6	130/100	110	7.295	37
	120–200	26.4	1580	29.7	124/ 90	116	7.201	37
b	40–75	24.0		21.4			7.231	38

We would like to express our thanks to Messrs. J. Pfrimmer + Co., 852 Erlangen, West Germany, for their support in carrying out our studies.

Our results underline the importance of an early commencement of fluid replacement, i.e. within one hour after trauma.

Oral substitution during volume deficiency

According to Rosenthal (5) and Fox (3), a volaemic shock can be controlled by peroral supply of electrolyte solutions. For our investigations we used Liquisorb[R] BW of J. Pfrimmer + Co., a modified Haldane solution with the following composition (Table 2).

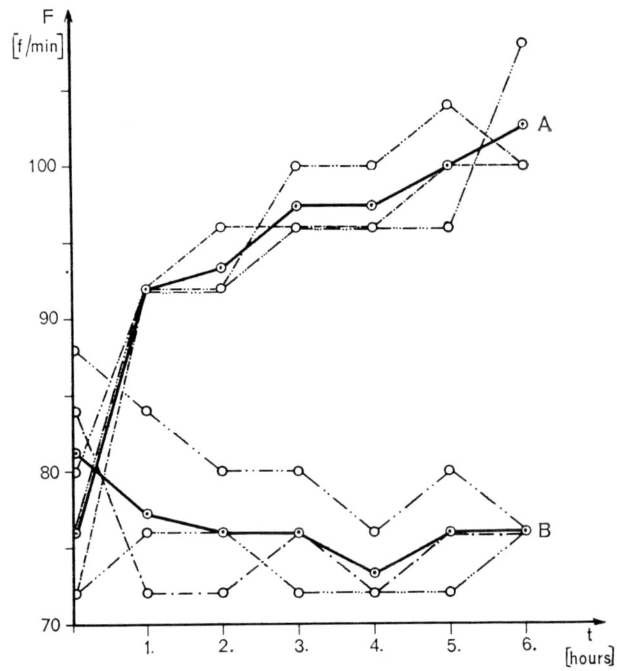

Fig. 1. Pulse rate (F) during artificial volume deficiency, healthy subjects. — a) without Liquisorb[R] BW. — b) with supply of Liquisorb[R] BW.

As you may recognize from the composition, it contains half quantities of electrolytes. The tolerance of the solution was examined on 50 normal subjects on two consecutive days.

1500 to 2000 ml of the electrolyte lemonade were drunk exclusively per day. Subjective

TABLE 2.

Composition of Liquisorb[R] BW

Na^+	60 mval/l	HCO_3—	28	mval/l
K^+	4 mval/l	Glucose	44	g/l
Ca^{++}	4 mval/l	Ascorbic acid	100	mg/l
Mg^{++}	4 mval/l	Lactoflavinphosphate	2,5	mg/l
Cl^-	44 mval/l	Nicotinamide	12	mg/l

intolerance symptoms were not observed. No deviations from the normal appeared in the serum and urine osmolality, in the haematocrit, standard bicarbonate or the pCO_2 of the arterial blood.

A 2/3 electrolyte solution is also tolerable and, if exclusively supplied, leaves the electrolyte metabolism in steady state. 10 subjects received this solution for 3 days ad libitum. Osmolality and ionogramme of the serum and the urine did not show any definite dependence on the amount supplied. Disturbances in haemodynamic regulation did not develop.

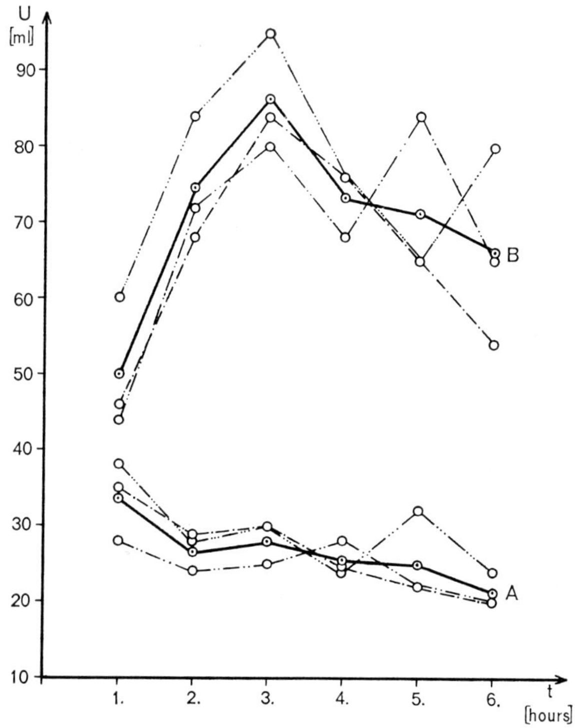

Fig. 2. Hourly urinary output (U) during artificial volume deficiency, healthy subjects. — a) without supply of Liquisorb[R] BW. — b) with supply of Liquisorb[R] BW.

In another series, 6 healthy persons were investigated to see if a shock prophylaxis was possible with a peroral substitution. After 12 hours of fasting, 15 per cent of the circulating volume were taken and 250 ml/hour of Liquisorb[R] BW were supplied for 6 hours (Fig. 1). The non-substituted control group developed symptoms of impending shock. One of them was the tachycardia which is shown in Fig. 1. The upper group of the curves corresponds to the pulse rate of the non-substituted test persons and the lower curves correspond to those being substituted. The differences in the pulse rate were evident after one hour and remained like that until the 6th hour. Furthermore, we observed in the non-substituted subjects a reduction in the blood pressure amplitude and an increase in haematocrit. Without substitution the urine production also decreased as you will clearly see in Fig. 2. The substituted persons showed normal urine output, whereas the non-substituted persons developed an oliguria.

It follows from these results that a shock prophylaxis during experimental volume deficits in healthy persons is possible by peroral supply of the afore-mentioned solution.

Oral substitution in burn patients

We have also used the peroral substitution successfully on shock exposed burn patients. 58 patients with 12 to 34 per cent burns of the body surface were admitted to hospital within one hour after their trauma. Only 4 of them could not drink the electrolyte lemonade. 16 of 23 patients, however, whose accident happened earlier, i.e. 1.5 to 3 hours earlier, were not able to drink the solution because of sickness, vomiting, centralisation of the circulation and unconsciousness.

We examined the gastro-intestinal absorptive capacity in another 10 patients with 12 to 26 per cent burns of the body surface. In the first hour after admission to the hospital, 1000 ml of Liquisorb[R] BW were given and in the second hour 750 ml in about 50 ml amounts. We controlled the passage of the electrolyte solution through the stomach with a stomach tube. The absorption of the solution was satisfactory in patients without centralisation of the circulation, but if a centralisation was existing, the absorption of the electrolyte lemonade was unsatisfactory. These patients were subsequently infused intravenously. After having re-established nearly normal circulatory conditions, we were then in the position to substitute perorally. A simple clinical test for the absorptive capacity of the intestine is the filling of the peripheral veins and the microcirculation of the skin as Folkow (2) has described it.

Our last experiment proved that after peroral substitution, the urine output of the burn patient is significantly higher than after intravenous infusion alone. First of all, the burn shock was met with intravenous infusion for 6 hours. After that, the patients received exclusively peroral Liquisorb[R] BW for another 6 hours and therewith produced an average of 41 ml urine per hour. In the next 6-hour-phase the patient's average excretion was 35 ml urine per hour during paranteral infusion exclusively. The urine output in the next 6 hours rose on the average to 40 ml per hour again while receiving peroral Liquisorb.

These results of an increased urine output after oral supply of a hypotonic electrolyte solution correspond to the animal experiments of Haberich et al. (4). These differences may be due to a primary osmotic receptor function of the liver.

With the present knowledge of the pathophysiology of burns, an immediate and adequate emergency treatment is mandatory (Ahnefeld, 1). We think on account of our investigations that the electrolyte lemonade Liquisorb[R] BW which we have developed is appropriate for shock prophylaxis in burn patients. If correctly indicated, the early use of it may prevent serious haemodynamic irregularities.

Indications

Indications for the use of Liquisorb[R] BW are among others:

1. shock prophylaxis immediately after the burn trauma until admission to hospital;
2. in hospital, for completing infusion therapy;
3. in disasters where there are great numbers of burn patients, as a temporary sole source of fluid replacement.

Contraindications

Clearly defined contraindications for the oral application of Liquisorb[R] BW are:
1. life-threatening volume deficiency and centralisation of the circulation;
2. vomiting, diarrhoea, trauma or stenosis of the gastro-intestinal tract;
3. psychomotoric states of agitation, somnolence, coma.

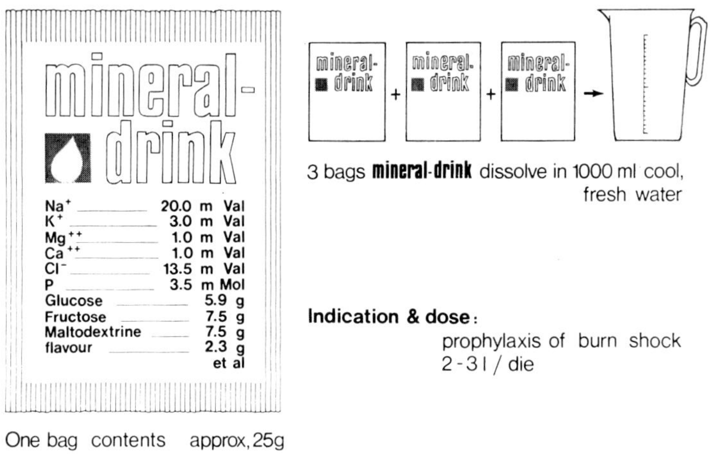

Fig. 3. The newest conception of an electrolyte lemonade (Mineraldrink[R]) for oral substitution therapy.

Finally, we want to present the new solution Mineraldrink[R] (Fig. 3) which has been developed by J. Pfrimmer + Co. on the basis of our investigations. Fig. 3 shows the composition of Mineraldrink[R] as well as recommendations for the preparation and dosage for burn patients.

Summary

At the end of the first hour, in a patient with moderate burns there is a 20 per cent deficit of the intravascular volume. This deficit can be reduced by the ingestion of a modified Haldane solution, the composition of which was decided upon after trials in healthy persons and moderately burned patients. When administered early and in sufficient amounts, this "electrolyte lemonade" can prevent shock for 3 to 6 hours. Renal function remains intact and the absorption of this solution is not disturbed in the early stages. This solution has many possibilities: as first aid before hospitalization of burn patients, in conjunction with intravenous therapy in burn patients, and in instances of mass traumatic injuries.

References

1. Ahnefeld, F. W. (1966): Die initiale Phase der Verbrennungskrankheit. Wehrdienst und Gesundheit, Darmstadt.
2. Folkow, B. (1962): Vom Nervensystem ausgehende Einflüsse auf die Strombahn unter besonderer Berücksichtigung der vasokonstriktorisch wirkenden Nervenfasern. In: Der Schock, Pathogenese und Therapie, Berlin, Göttingen, Heidelberg, 69.

3. Fox, Ch. L. (1944): Oral sodium lactate in the treatment of burn shock. J. Amer. med. Ass. 124 : 207.
4. Haberich, F. J. (1972): Osmorezeptoren im Portalkreislauf und ihre Bedeutung für die Regulation des Wasserhaushaltes. Triangel 4 : 123.
5. Rosenthal, S. M. (1943): Experimental chemotherapy of burns and shock. V. Therapy with rum and sodium salts. Publ. Health Rep. 58 : 1429.

F. W. A., Dept. of Anaesthesiology,
University of Ulm,
7900 Ulm, F.R.G.

MODIFIED GELATINE AND POLYVINYLPYRROLIDONE FOR VOLUME REPLACEMENT IN EXTENSIVE BURNS — A COMPARATIVE STUDY

K. M. DURRANI

Plastic Surgery and Burns Service, Civil Hospital and Dow Medical College, Karachi, Pakistan

INTRODUCTION

Extravasation of plasma-like fluid following acute thermal injury lasts for about 48 hours, at the end of which period the sequestered fluid begins to re-enter the vascular compartment. About this very time infection begins to gain a foothold and may be quite well established by the fifth day.

In studies of resuscitation aimed at evaluating various replacement fluids for the shock phase, observations of physiological parameters during the first 2 days are particularly significant, since alterations of hemodynamic status are not yet adulterated by many other complicating factors of later stages. With time, burn pathophysiology changes its character from one of pure hemodynamic-heat-regulation disturbance to one where multiple hostile forces interact to destroy the organism. After the 5th day, the picture certainly is far from one of pure hypovolemia.

This paper is a report of observations on two colloids used in acute burns during the resuscitative phase, covering a period of five days from start of treatment.

MATERIAL AND METHODS

Sixty consecutive burn cases admitted to the Burn Service were randomly assigned to one of the two colloids at the ratio of 3 : 2. The first colloid was a 3.5 per cent solution of a degraded gelatine polymer containing 0.85 per cent NaCl and some other ions (Haemaccel, Hoechst-molecular weight 35,000) while the other was a 4 per cent solution, of polyvinylpyrrolidone (a formaldehyde polymer) containing 0.7 per cent NaCl (Periston Bayer — molecular weight 30,000).

On admission, the extent of the burn was estimated according to the rule of nines (3). Depth was assessed clinically and "net third degree burn" calculated from this by halving the second degree extent and adding to the third degree figure (1). Intravenous (I/V) fluid therapy was then worked out according to the Brooke Army formula which prescribes a ratio of 1 : 3 between colloids and electrolytes (5). Burns above 50 percent net third degree were regarded the same as 50 percent burns.

All burns were treated closed and treatment remained strictly similar except for the I/V colloid being tested. Serial observations were made during the next 5 days on the following parameters:

Clinical: Pulse, blood pressure (b.p.), peripheral venous pressure (v.p.), temperature, respiration, urinary output, sensorium and weight.

Laboratory: Hematocrit (Hct), hemoglobin (Hb), RBC count, platelet count, blood urea nitrogen (BUN), serum electrolytes, blood specific gravity (sp.gr.), bleeding time (B.T.), clotting time (C.T.), urine sp. gr. and electrolyte content of 24-hour specimens.

RESULTS

36 cases fell in group I (Haemaccel) and 24 in group II (Periston). The groups were quite similar in average age, body weight and total extent of burns. Female sex predominated in both groups but particularly so in group II (Table 1).

TABLE 1

Basic Data

Group Identification	I	II
Colloid used	Hematocrit	Periston
No. of cases	36	24
Age (years)	20.2	22.1
Weight (kg)	37.9	40.5
Extent of burn per cent body surface 2nd + 3rd degrees	53.0	50.6
Female : Male	1.2 : 3.0	

TABLE 2

Amount and type of Intravenous Fluids

Type of Fluid	Amount of Fluid (ml/kg/ per cent burn)	
	Group I	Group II
Colloids and Electrolytes	3.3	3.3
5 per cent Dextrose in water	4.0	4.0
Total for study period	7.3	7.3

Actual I/V fluids received during the period of study averaged the same in both groups (Table 2). No colloids other than the two under study were administered during this period.

Clinical parameters:

Pulse, temperature and respiration curves ran fairly parallel with each other (Fig. 1). In group I, these curves were seen to rise until the 3rd day and then showed a more gradual fall until the end of the study period. In contrast, group II revealed a rise throughout the study period, albeit the rate of rise slowed down midway through this period. The mean daily temperature remained about half degree F lower in group II compared with group I throughout the 5-day period.

Blood pressure and venous pressure: There was no difference between the two groups in respect of these parameters (Fig. 2, 3). Both factors came within the normal range soon after start of treatment and remained so subsequently.

Urinary outputs followed the same pattern as blood pressure and remained satisfactory — around 1,200 ml/24 hours in group I and 1,000 ml/24 hours in group II from the 2nd day onwards (Fig. 4).

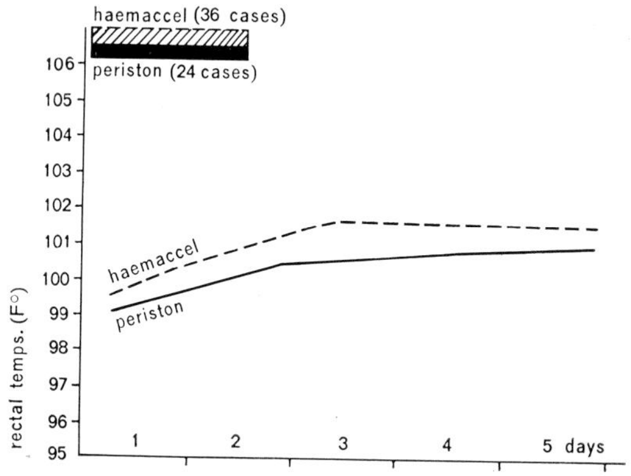

Fig. 1. Mean temperatures (ordinate, in Fahrenheit)

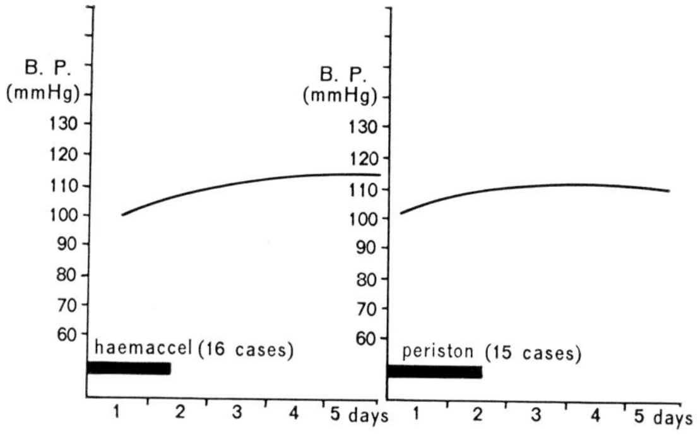

Fig. 2. Mean blood pressures (in mmHg)

Disturbed sensorium on any occasion during the study period was noticed twice as often in group I (42 per cent of cases) as in group II (21 per cent of cases). No correlation of this could be demonstrated with BUN, high fever (above 103 degrees F, rectal) or with serum electrolyte levels.

Laboratory parameters:

Hematocrit (Fig. 5). Group II had a more rapid and greater fall in Hct compared to group I. Hb, RBC and platelet counts followed closely the Hct curve in both groups.

Bleeding and clotting times (Fig. 6). Prolongation of B.T. was noted in both groups with start of treatment. On the 2nd and 3rd day, group II remained stationary while group I rose after a short-lived drop. On the 4th and 5th days B.T. fell in both groups. C.T. followed approximately the same course as B.T. of the respective group.

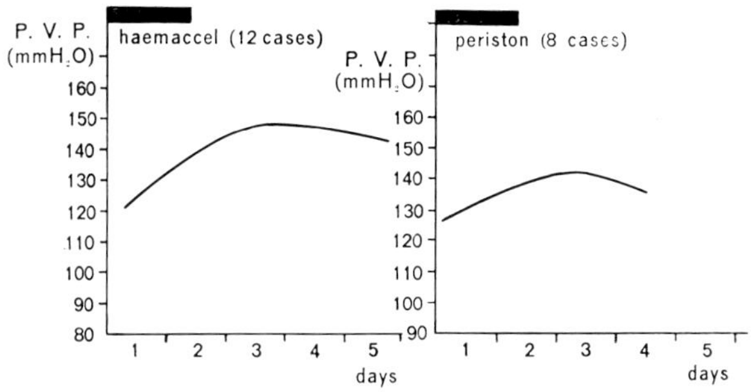

Fig. 3. Peripheral venous pressures (PVP, in mmH_2O)

Blood sp. gr. Falling sp. gr. was observed in 63.1 per cent of group I and 66.6 per cent of group II cases immediately following establishment of treatment. The rest of the cases showed either a rise in sp. gr. or it remained unchanged inspite of treatment.

Urine sp. gr. and electrolyte excretion. As an index of adequate kidney

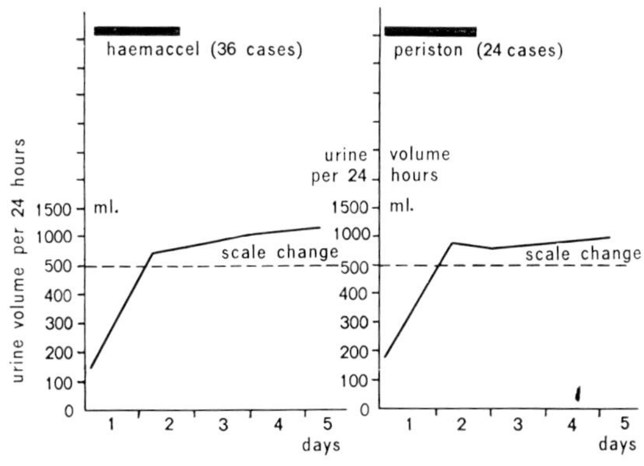

Fig. 4. Mean urinary outputs per 24 hours

perfusion, normal or low (1010) urine sp. gr. on the second day or thereafter was noted in over 90 per cent of cases in both the groups. Adequate electrolyte excretion was observed more often in group II: 78.5 per cent of cases of this group had adequate Na and 85.7 per cent adequate K excretion as compared with 66.6 per cent and 77.7 per cent respectively of group I.

BUN and serum electrolytes. BUN above 45 mgm/100 ml on any one day of study was noted in 27.3 per cent of group I and 33.3 per cent of group II cases. Thus a larger percentage of group I cases remained within the normal range.

No consistent pattern was observed in serum electrolyte levels of either group following treatment.

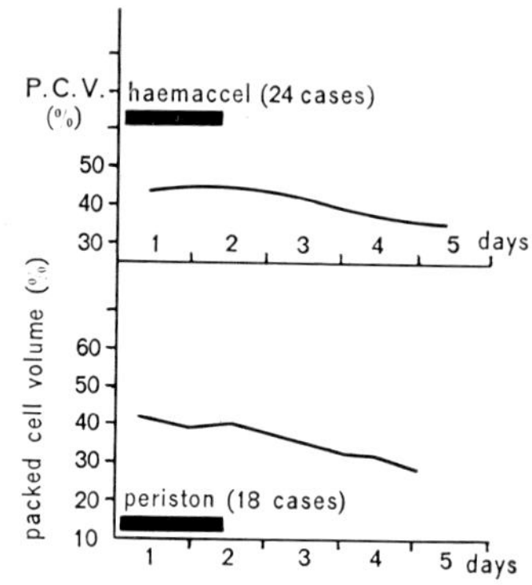

Fig. 5. Mean haematocrit values (in per cent)

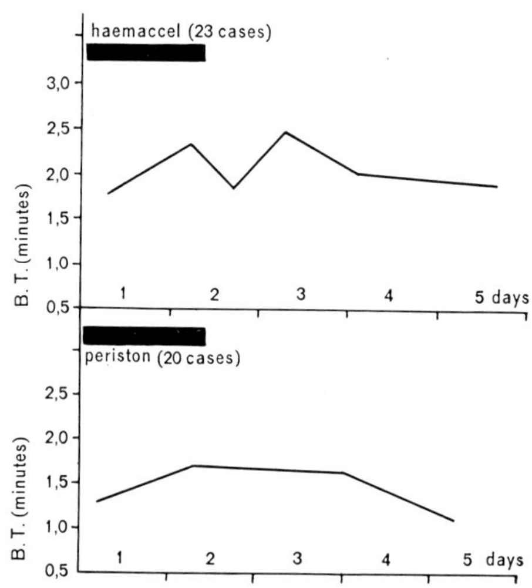

Fig. 6. Mean bleeding times (in min.)

Mortality Figures:

48-hour mortality was 36.1 per cent in group I and 37.5 percent in group II. 5-day mortality was 61.2 and 62.5 per cent respectively. No remarkable difference was observed between survival rates of the two groups. In 13 very extensive burns (above 70 per cent body surface), 8 in group I and 5 in group II, 50 per cent were alive at the end of 48 hours and 25 percent at the end of 72 hours in group I and only 20 per cent at 48 hours and none at 72 hours in group II. One person in group I (12.5 per cent) was still alive at the end of 5 days.

Compared with Moyer's plasma series (1953), group I showed a better survival and group II worse survival.

Submitted to Bull and Fisher's grid analysis technique (2), the ratio of observed mortality to expected mortality was 1.09 for group I and 1.12 for group II, i.e. slightly higher in group II but not significantly different from that in I.

Conclusion

Both the colloids tested were able to sustain adequate hemodynamic functions in acute thermal burns of average extent 50 per cent body surface, when administered according to Brooke Army formula, in over 50 per cent of cases during a period of 5 days. Five-day survival was less than 40 per cent in either group, with little difference between the two. In burns of 70 per cent body surface or larger, modified gelatine preparation proved more efficacious than the formaldehyde derivative in prolonging survival.

References

1. Artz, C. P. and Moncrief, J. A. (1969): The Treatment of Burns, 2nd Edition. Philadelphia, Saunders.
2. Bull, J. P. and Fisher, A. J. (1954): A study of mortality in a burn unit: a revised estimate. Ann. Surg. 139: 269.
3. Kyle, M. J. and Wallace, A. B. (1951): Fluid replacement in burnt children. Brit. J. plast. Surg. 3 : 194.
4. Moyer, C. A. (1953): An assessment of the therapy of burns: A clinical study. Ann. Surg. 137 : 628.
5. Reiss, E., Stirman, J. A., Artz, C. P., Davis, J. H. et al. (1953): Fluid and electrolyte balance in burns. J. Amer. med. Ass. 152 : 1309.

K. M. D., Plastic Surgery and Burns Service, Civil Hospital, Karachi, Pakistan

RECOMMENDATION FOR A CLINICAL CONCEPT BASED ON EXPERIMENTAL DATA FOR INITIAL TREATMENT OF THE BURN SHOCK

A. BERGER, F. FINSETH, M. MAZUR and J. F. BURKE

Department of Plastic and Reconstructive Surgery, First Surgical Clinic, Vienna, Austria and General Hospital, Harvard Medical School, Boston, Mass. 02114, U.S.A.

The immediate post-burn period is marked by changes in the dynamics of the circulations and capillary fluid shift which are called the burn shock. A lot of papers have been published containing studies of the first post-burn period (1, 2, 5, 6). An important feature of this disturbance is the change in capillary permeability (2). For studying the capillary fluid transport phenomenon, we designed a perfusion model (4). First we tried to clear up this model and secondly we studied the dynamic changes immediately after deep second and third degree burns, and possibilities of influencing the immediate post-burn period with cristalloids, colloids or plasma.

METHOD AND MATERIAL

A preparation of skin, muscles and bones from a backside of a guinea pig is used. The animal is eviscerated and the aorta and v. cava cannulated. The tubes are connected to a membrane oxygenator (Fig. 1). Venous and arterial pressures, temperature and weight are continuously recorded. pH, pCO_2, Hct and protein and electrolyte are examined at certain intervals by micromethods. Changes of the weight of the preparation express changes in the capillary fluid transport (7). This model could be kept under physiological conditions for 4 hours. A mathematical model (Mazur) is used to explain the reactions, especially the weight and pressure changes in our studies. An exponential equation expresses the weight change — $Y = A(1 - e^{-Bt}) + Ct$. Resistance is calculated by using Ohm's law and adapting it to fluid mechanics. Energy is also calculated by using a computer program.

The ideal reaction can be therefore forecast and the differences can be studied between the experiment and these data. A reproducible burn mark was administered to the backside of the animal at the range of 20 per cent of the perfused surface. The average weight of the experimental animals in this study was 400 g. For the burn mark an acrylic mask was used and the animal was brought into contact with boiling water (90 degrees of centigrade) for 30 or 10 seconds. The extravasation and deposit was tested using J^{131} labelled human albumin. The main data can be seen in Table 1. The data were analysed by using the above-mentioned model adapted to these special problems.

TABLE 1.

Main data of our perfusion model using burn marks 20 p. c. BSA.

t 0–180	control	20 p. c. burn	lactated Ringer	Addition of	
				Dextran 70	Plasma
Diff. Wg	+ 0.61	+ 5.15	+ 3.76	+ 3.97	+ 4.36
Resistance R Torr. min/ml	0.015	1.025	0.149	0.227	0.476
Plasma activity J^{131} per cent	1.21	2.10	1.45	1.32	1.46
Skin per cent dry/wet	67.3	77.2	85.3	72.9	75.1
Muscle per cent dry/wet	73.8	80.1	74.0	80.8	81.6
Skin deposit	0.0071	0.0108	0.0737	0.0157	0.0251
Muscle deposit	0.0075	0.0066	0.0243	0.0283	0.0075
Potassium diff.	+ 3.38	+ 4.47	+ 3.27	+ 5.51	+ 4.47
Natrium diff.	— 2.60	— 7.10	+ 0.50	— 6.20	+ 9.60
Protein concentr.	+ 0.92	+ 0.89	+ 0.47	+ 0.11	+ 0.38
pH	7.40	7.35	7.28	7.27	7.42

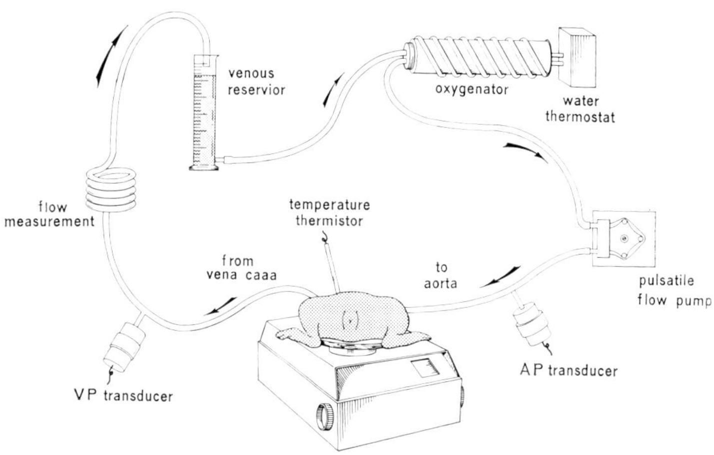

Fig. 1. Experimental model using the backside of guinea pig for perfusion.

Eight different experimental groups were used.

Group 1: 30 second burn, 20 p.c. BSA;

Group 2: 30 second burn, 20 p.c. BSA, 30 minutes after setting the burn mark, lactated Ringer 3.0 ml/p.c. BSA/kg/24 h was added;

Group 3: 30 second burn, 20 p.c. BSA, 30 minutes later 6 p.c. Dextran 70 was given using the formula 1.0 ml/p.c. BSA/kg/24 h;

Group 4: 30 second burn, 20 p.c. BSA, 30 minutes later homologous plasma was given intravenously.

The same program, but only 10 seconds burning, was repeated in group 5 to 8.

As can be seen in the diagram (Fig. 2), a typical first peak of weight gain can be observed after 30 minutes, a second about 120 and a third 180 minutes after burn. Resistance in the controls showed a marked increase. The lymphatics were dilated (1) and, with Risa, extravasation could be observed also far from the burn mark. The groups treated with colloids or plasma showed similar curves as the controls, group 2 showed significant

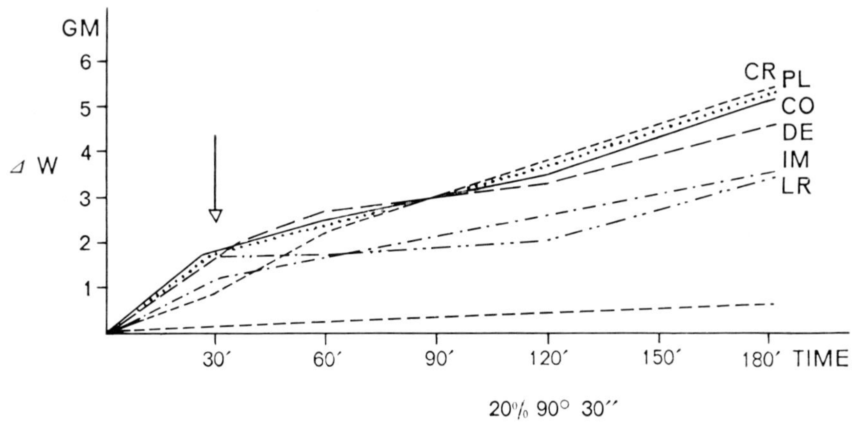

Fig. 2. Weight changes after burn and under treatment with cristalloids, colloids and plasma (W — weight, CR — hydrocortison, PL — homologous plasma, CO — control, DE — 6 per cent Dextran — 70, IM — indomethacin, LR — lactated Ringer)

differences in weight and also in the autoradiographic studies. The stable state could be reached very quickly and in the specimens a marked oedema and signs of rapid fluid transport could be observed. Group 5 to 8 showed only slight differences so that these groups need not be discussed.

Discussion

If we try to draw conclusions on the basis of our experiments, but in connection with recent papers such as Moncrief's, the following program can be recommended as being at present the optimum treatment for the first post burn period after severe burns: In the first 6 hours, the best solution for regaining a stable haemodynamic state are the cristalloids. Colloids and plasma are lost in the extravascular space and, consequently, more fluid passes into the inactive damaged tissues. But after this period, colloidosmotic active substances are again needed in the vascular compartement for building up a new stable state in this field as well. A major factor is also the increasing oedema under the cristalloid therapy. This is why local damage may increase if using only one type of therapy. If the burn shock situation is treated well and this is possible when using values of central venous pressure, urine output and astrup, the blood pattern should be normalized. Electrolytes must be administered and especially plasma, but this is well known. But using this concept with the help or the guidelines offered by a computer program calculating also the energy balance, can make also critical cases survive, and such a disadvantage as increasing local damage caused by the necessary initial therapy can be avoided.

In this short time at disposal it was only possible to raise a certain number of problems for useful discussion and future investigation.

References

1. Arturson, G. (1971): Evaporation and fluid replacement. In: Research in Burns. Huber-Verlag, Bern, 520.
2. Berger, A., Burke, J. F., Finseth, F., Mazur, M. and Billote, J. B. (1972): Zur Dynamik des kapillaren Flüssigkeitstransportes. Kongressbericht Österr. Chir. Kongr.
3. Burke, J. F. (1968): A critical survey of the conventional principles of general therapy during the first phase of burns and prospects of new trends. Present Clin. Aspects of Burns, Maribor, 29.
4. Finseth, F., Hattori, H. and Burke, J. F. (1972): Perfusion of an isolated capillary system for the analysis of capillary transport phenomena. J. Trauma 12 : 75.
5. Moncrief, J. A. (1973): Burns, Medical Progress. New Engl. J. Med. 288 : 444.
6. Polk, H. C. Jr. and Linder, S. Van (1971): Saline solutions for burn shock resuscitation, an experimental dissection of its elements. Research in Burns, Huber-Verlag, Bern, 75.
7. Pappenheimer, J. R. (1953): Passage of molecules through capillary walls. Physiol. Rev. 33 : 387.

A. B., 1st Surgical Clinic,
Alserstrasse 4,
1090 Wien, Austria

THERAPEUTIC ROLE OF ESCHARECTOMIES IN THE PERIOD OF BURN SHOCK

Z. JANŽEKOVIČ

General Hospital, Maribor, Yugoslavia

Nowadays, it is no problem to control shock, and the fight against infection has become more successful. However, we still lose severe burns in spite of all our efforts. The unsolved problems seem to paralyse the enthusiasm of those concerned with the treatment of burns, who would like to possess a more understandable explanation of the essence of terrible events caused by burning.

The clinical results obtained by primary necrectomies in extensive deep burns justify the conclusion that more of our efforts should be concentrated towards an earlier and more adequate treatment in the early postburn phase.

Such treatment has not only the advantage of shortening the burn disease, but also improves the defense mechanism of the body during the infection phase.

Primary necrectomy is in our opinion indicated in all deep burns over 50 p.c. of the body surface. In critical cases an exchange transfusion should precede the necrectomy.

Material and methods

In the past years primary necrectomy was performed in our Unit in 9 patients, who suffered from burns involving up to 70 p.c. of the body surface. In adults 15 to 20 p.c. of the burned surface was excised in one operation, in children 40 to 60 p.c.

During the first operation, preference was given to excise deep burns in functional areas and dermal burns, which were then covered by homografts, which assure final epithelisation of the areas concerned.

As deep burns, we considered all those where no blood return could be observed on pressure.

Excised areas of the head and of the hands were covered by autografts, whenever possible, other areas of the body by fresh homografts.

The excision was performed as usually by horizontal cuts using blades of the Humby knife, which were fixed on an improvised handle. The excised areas of the extremities were covered while the tourniquet was still in place, all other excised areas were covered by grafts after the bleeding had stopped.

A metal wool compressive dressing was applied in all cases, serving at the same time also as an adequate and comfortable immobilisation. Whenever necessary, the excision was performed circumferentially and it was found that the pressure of the body against the bed did not interfere with the take of the grafts.

The excision was technically easier and quicker if performed early, because of the initial oedema. The loss of blood was relatively small; it was measured by weighing and replaced immediately. During the operation the electrolyte and acid base balance was checked and corrected accordingly.

The anaesthesia lasted from 4 to 6 hours, the operation itself from 1.5 to 4 hours, depending on the depth, localisation and extent of the burned area.

In a few instances necrectomy was indicated on the second or the third day because of persisting shock. In one case of a 60 p.c. subdermal burn, admitted in a critical condition, first an exchange transfusion and incisions of the necrotic areas were performed, followed by radical necrectomy and application of homografts 12 hours later.

The first dressing was done in all cases after 24 hours in order to check the situation.

The second excision was done the fourth postburn day, i.e. still during the optimal period before the possible onset of infection.

Results

All pathological symptoms disappeared at the end of the operation.

All patients except one (a 70 per cent burnt child, which died on the 52nd day), treated by primary necrectomy survived and were healed in a period of time related to the severity and extension of the burned area. The severity of infection was reduced, following the second excision performed the third or the fourth day and the amount of the infection still existing was very well tolerated by all patients. The grafts took well and the donor areas were healed in eight to ten days. An increase of the body weight was registered in all patients on the day they left the hospital.

Discussion

The essence of the quick decrease of the morbidity observed after primary necrectomy can be explained by the sequence of events, occurring during the operative procedure.

The factors influencing these changes are: a good anaesthesia, which improves the oxygenation of the patient; the decrease of the burned surface; the exchange of blood; the reduced escape of fluids after the resorption of oedema in the excised areas, which were immediately covered by grafts.

In the classical type of treatment, as applied to the burn wound under anaesthesia, no improvement of this kind can be noted.

In extensive burns in adults the burned surface was reduced from 60 to 40 p.c. in the first operation. This means, that the remaining burned areas were sufficiently large to maintain the body in a pathological state. Even so, a great improvement of the general condition of the patient could be observed after the first excision.

We must, therefore, concentrate on the events connected with the escape of intravascular fluids, which has a similar effect as the control of bleeding in a haemorrhagic shock, and the effect obtained by the change of blood.

The study of morphological alterations in burns of various depth in different postburn periods brings into evidence interesting changes in particular tissues. The tissue elements show reversible and irreversible changes. The primary gradual decrease of their intensity is accompanied by characteristic changes of the vessels, which are different in the arterial and venous network of the circulation. In the livid areas of contracted capillaries and thrombosed veins undamaged strong arterioles can be found. Livid areas mean partial or complete venous blocking of the circulation. Therefore, the pressure in the intact arterioles increases. This sudden resistance influences on one side the blood pressure and on the other side the pressure against the damaged endothelium, causing thus the intervascular fluids to escape into the extravascular space.

The influence of the heat can be felt also in the vessels, situated proximally to the capillary network. The capillaries and the subcutaneous veins may be contracted, dilated or thrombosed. The oedema, arising in the areas situated proximally i.e. in the neighbouring non-burned areas, may be also explained as due to stasis, occurring in the regions of the functionally insufficient venous trunk. Stasis is, therefore, the third factor, which in the presence of damaged vessels, the increased pressure in the intact arterioles and the existing venous block, influences the development of oedema in the burned area.

The changes in the vessels can be best observed in contact burns. In performing horizontal excision, all the above-mentioned changes can be found in the subcutaneous and surrounding tissues, even if the clinical aspect of the skin in the area is intact. This means, no doubt, that the heat affects the blood and the lymphatic fluid circulating through the burned area and, therefore, also the neighbouring tissues.

In the damaged venous blood, which flows through the burned area next to altered blood elements, toxic protein fractions and an increased number of enzymes can be found. The difference of the temperature in the blood stream before and after the burn may amount 3 to 4 degrees of centigrade.

Due to the increase of the temperature and the alterations of the biochemical properties, the burned blood represents a new dimension of damage, which is instantaneous and complex. The anatomical and functional integrity of the endothelium is destroyed locally and in distant areas. The damaged endothelium, which affects the whole biological potential of the extravascular space, influences also the function of differentiated cells in distant organs and is more marked in organs containing a rich blood network.

In the chaotic situation caused by the interaction of all those alterations, the whole stability and defence capacity of the body is affected.

The intensity and extent of the damage to the endothelium depends on the intensity of the thermal effect, the length of its duration and the area affected.

The alterations of the endothelium and of the blood affect also the distribution of the blood elements in the circulation. Normal erythrocytes are blocked in the altered plasma and blood elements in the central part of the vessels. This state of affairs affects also the oxygenation.

It should therefore be our task to normalize the quality and the quantity of the blood. This would lessen the load on the damaged endothelium and accelerate its regeneration.

It is, therefore, not enough to fill up the intravascular space, to infuse blood, but also to change it partially or completely, depending on the intensity of the damage.

By performing a primary necrectomy, the following advantages are obtained:

1. we change a noticeable amount of blood, by which the oxygenating capacity increases, the toxic factors of the blood become diluted, and the restitution of the endothelium accelerates.
2. in the excised areas we eliminate the blocked part of the venous circulation and so the escape of fluids from the vessels is decreased.

Conclusion

In view of the blocked venous circulation from the burned area and the decreasing intensity of shock (even without adequate therapy), it is difficult to explain the resorption of toxins from the burned tissues. The release of enzymes and pathological fractions of proteins into the venous stream immediately after burning, and morphological alterations of the vessels, justify the hypothesis of a burn of the blood and its consecutive action on the endothelium.

A quicker restitution of the endothelium can be obtained by changing the blood and by excluding the blocked venous vessels through a partial excision, diminishing at the same time the escape of fluids into the extravascular space. The regenerative power of organs becomes thus increased and this affects essentially also the defense potential of the body.

We consider, therefore, that the clinical results obtained so far justify primary necrectomy as an important weapon in the therapeutic program of the early postburn period.

References

1. JACKSON, M. D. (1969): Second thoughts on the burn wound. J. Trauma 9 : 839.
2. JANŽEKOVIČ, Z. (1968): In: Present Clinical Aspects of Burns: a Symposium. Ed. by M. Derganc. Č. P. Mariborski tisk, Maribor, 99.
3. JANŽEKOVIČ, Z. (1970): A new concept in the early excision and immediate grafting of burns. J. Trauma 10 : 1103.

Z. J., Vinarska 10B,
6200 Maribor, Yugoslavia

HYPERBARIC OXYGEN THERAPY IN THIRD DEGREE BURN WOUNDS — A MICROANGIOGRAPHIC STUDY

J. HAERTWIG

Department of Surgery, University of Freiburg i. Br., F.R.G.

In order to test the effect of intermittent hyperbaric oxygen therapy we examined 100 albino rats with third degree burns by microangiography. The angiography was done according to the method of Schlesinger. After anesthesia and heparinization the contrast media consisting of 4 per cent gelatine, 10 per cent formalin and Micropaque was perfused into the animals over a nylon catheter inserted in the aorta over 10 min. under a pressure of 120 cm H_2O. This solution fills vessels up to a radius of 20/μ after perfusion and becomes firm after 15 minutes. After excision of the back skin radiography was performed using a special film (industrial X-Ray Type single coated). For this purpose a surface therapy X-ray machine RT 100 from Müller was used. Using the microangiograms we tried to find the best method for a standard burn on 40 rats. In ether anesthesia a copper plate of 11 sq. cm with a pressure of 300 pond at 250 degrees of centigrade was used in application times between 1 and 25 seconds after shaving of the back skin. After 15 seconds at 300 pond and 250 degrees of centigrade we found no more vessels in the angiograms. Longer times of burn lead to a burn of the back musculature. These results confirm examinations of Schönenberger and Allgöwer. In our further experiments we used 100 rats of 300 grs weight with a standardized burn with 250 degrees of centigrade under 300 ponds pressure in an application time of 15 sec. 50 animals served as controls. The other 50 were treated 3 times daily for 60 minutes with a hyperbaric chamber. The isobaric compression lasted 60 minutes at 2.5 ata. Compression and decompression were done with 0.2 kp/sq. cm/min, the treatment was continued for 28 days. Starting on the 14th day, every 2 days 6 animals of each group were examined by microangiography. The non-revascularized area was measured exactly planimetrically according to Perrins and Barmeyer. The revascularized area was the difference between the area of burn and the measured area which was not revascularized.

In the angiograms of the OHP treated animals 50 per cent of the burned area was revascularized after 14 days, versus only 17 per cent revascularized area in the control groups, which in addition showed distinct edema and inflammatory signs. The untreated group reached 85 per cent revascularized area after 26 days. The treated group reached this result already on the 20th day.

In this experiment using microangiographic studies we found a positive effect of intermittent hyperbaric oxygen therapy on the speed of revascularization of 3rd degree burns. In the treated group we found hardly any edema or inflammatory reaction of the burned area. The fluid loss from the burn wounds was smaller in the treated group in comparison to the control group. The faster regeneration under elevated partial oxygen pressure is explained by an increased rate of mitosis from Bullough and Ikeda. The point of action is unknown today. The steps of wound healing appeared up to 6 days earlier in the treated group versus the control group. In the treated group the capillaries of the wound edges started to grow faster towards the center of the burn than in the control group, and the connection to bigger vessels starts earlier. The wound area filled quickly with a distinct pattern of vascularization, while in the control group quality and quantity of the vascular pattern stayed far behind the treated group. These factors naturally could not be quantitatively differentiated in the evaluation of the microangiograms.

The separation of the sloughs started much earlier under the influence of oxygen therapy. By early debridement the favourable influence of oxygen therapy could be further improved, since the formation of wet chambers and abscesses under the sloughs can be avoided.

The removal of the sloughs was not done in our experiments in order not to disturb the standardization of the experiment. Systematic microscopical examinations of the lungs of the animals which had been treated with intermittent OHP showed no pathological changes.

J. H., Hugstetterstr. 55,
7800 Freiburg i.Br., F.R.G.

THE VALUE OF HYPER-PRESSURE-OXYGEN IN THE TREATMENT OF BURN DISEASE

Š. ŠIMKO, J. BLÁHA and I. JUGENBURG

Department for Burns and Reconstructive Surgery, Works Hospital, Košice-Šaca, Czechoslovakia

In this paper we report about the possibilities of applying Hyper-Pressure-Oxygen in the treatment of burns. We tried to find out the best way of using Hyper-Pressure-Oxygen (HPO) in burns and we shall recommend, on the basis of our best clinical experience in which way HPO therapy can be used.

We do not deal with the physiological basis of HPO generally.

We have been using individual small chambers since 1965. We worked with six one-man chambers, of which five were home-made and the last is a Dräger one-man chamber from Lübeck (Fig. 1a, b). Three of them were used in experimental practice and the other in clinics. In the treatment of burns we used exclusively the Dräger chamber. We had 4135 sessions, 435 sessions in burns treatment, in 85 burned patients.

After studying literature about clinical, experimental and theoretical possibilities of HPO in shock treatment, we supposed that HPO therapy could be very successful in the shock of the burned. We based this on the similarity of the hypovolaemic-haemorrhagic shock with the shock of the burned. We concluded that HPO is a very good and efficient way of treating hypovolaemic-haemorrhagic shock, but the burn shock seems to be a different question. Therefore we started some experiments rather complicated by the correct selection of the experimental animal, with regard to the oxygen used and the standard methods of producing burns. The results of our experiments were not such as to support the use of HPO in the treatment of the burn shock. We could not prove any significant benefit in the survival of our animals after burning.

Nevertheless we used HPO in 37 acutely burned patients, with burns covering over 50 p.c. of the body surface, in addition to the other classical methods of treatment. We used 2 ATA hyperpressure, never for longer than one-and-a-half hour of hyper-pressure once in 24 hours, using oxygen atmosphere. We repeated the sessions for a maximum of three days in succession in cases which seemed to be suitable.

We used in burned patients exclusively the Dräger chamber to our greatest satisfaction and until today we had more than 1000 hours of work without trouble. The possibility of assisted ventilation regulated from outside and monitoring are the great advantages of this type of chamber. But we had to overcome the problem of applying infusion therapy parallel with HPO. Our infusion sets are good up to 1/5 ATA, but above this

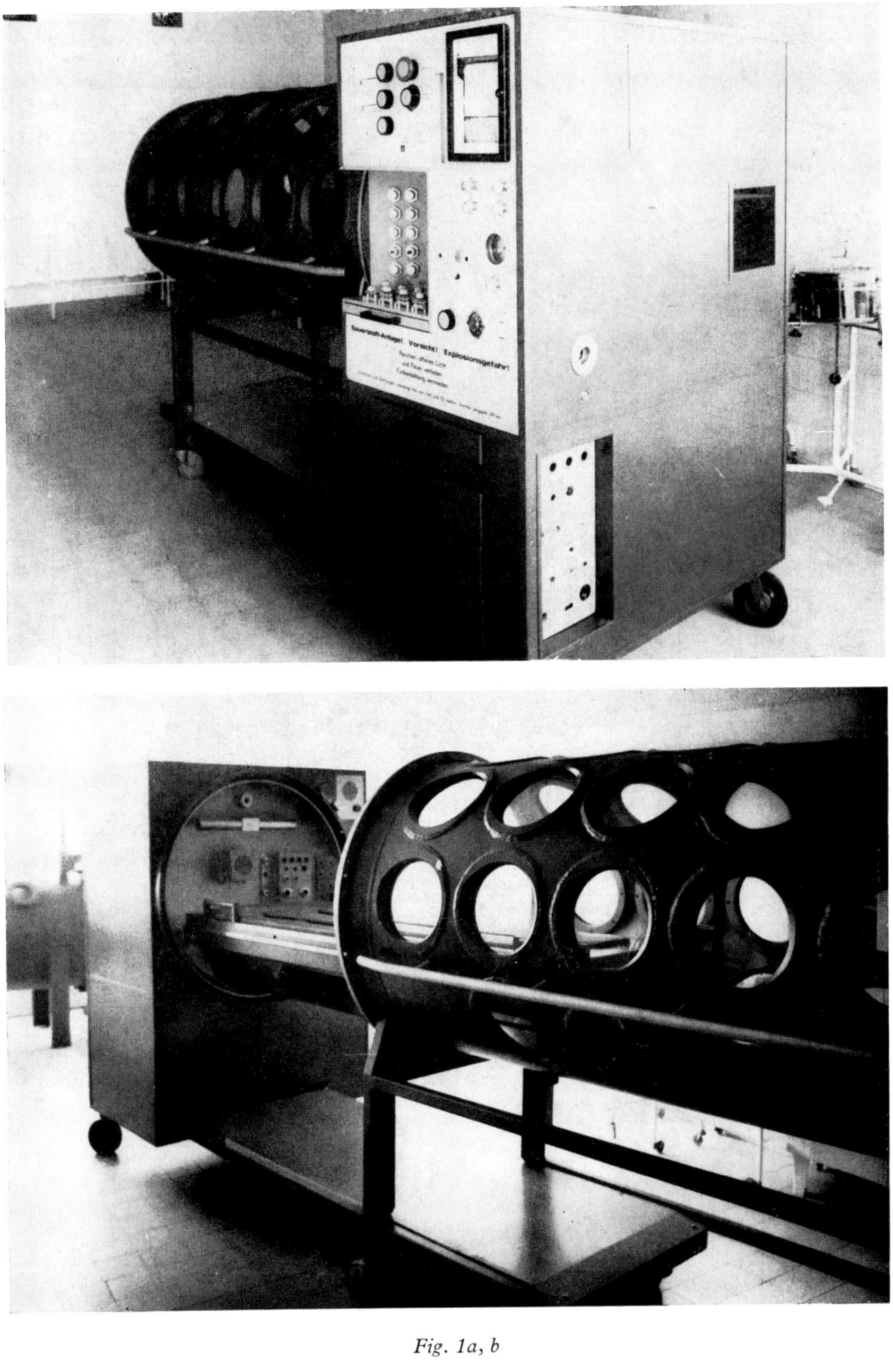

Fig. 1a, b

they are leaking. We solved this by using the pressure infusion as proposed by Bařinka from Brno to our greatest satisfaction, and so we used infusion therapy parallel to HPO.

In this clinical trial we found that HPO was not useful in the treatment of shock generally, but profitable in cases with confusion, unconsciousness and finally in burns combined with CO intoxications. High levels of COHb showed to be a further finding which should be followed routinely. Our department is part of the Works Hospital of the East Slovakian Iron Works where burns are very often combined with CO intoxication. We can prove that a surprisingly high percentage of our early dying patients showed high COHb levels (30 p.c. and higher). So we concluded that CO intoxications with a high level of COHb should be regarded as a bad prognostic sign. The application of HPO was also successful in some specific situations of electric burns. In 26 cases out of 37 we had the impression that HPO was very useful, because the treatment of these patients made a better start for further treatment. In the remaining 11 cases HPO was of no value.

Concluding, we can say that HPO showed to be a good adjuvans to the classic intravenous therapy in the first stage of burns disease (first 3 days) in the following cases:

- in burns with psychological disorders — 5 cases,
- in combination with CO intoxication, with COHb levels higher than 30 p.c. — 9 cases,
- in electric burns: with unconsciousness — 5 cases,
  with necroses and/or gangrene — 7 cases.

HPO proved to be not valuable in burns:

- of the respiratory tract — 5 cases,
- of small children younger than 10 years, with burned body surface over 50 p.c. — 6 cases.

We used HPO in 48 cases of burns in the second phase of burn disease. In this stage we face the problems of transplantation, covering the defects, infection, septicaemia and restitution of physical and mental power for complete recovery.

Early covering of the burned surface, freed from necrosis, is the basis of successful treatment of burns. This is why all methods which speed up the healing of transplants and secure transplantations are of great value for the treatment of burns disease.

We shall now examine the theoretical and experimental conditions permitting to use HPO in transplantation and in burns on the basis of our experimental and clinical trials and also on the basis of some papers read at the last 4th Hyperbaric Medical Congress in Sapporo.

Injured skin is restored primarily by migration of cells from the epidermis around the edges of the wound and cut surfaces of hair follicles and ducts of sweat glands. The time required for the epidermis to cover completely the wound surface, depends primarily on the speed at which the cells move and the distance between adjacent sources of epidermal cells. It must be noticed that it is active movement of the cells — they are not pushed by the pressure of mitoses at the wound edges. It is known that the hair follicles in young large white pigs are on average about 2 mm apart; the epidermal sheets migrating from adjacent follicles consequently travel about 1 mm until they unite, the epithelisation of the wound is completed in six days, and we can therefore deduce that epidermal cells cross the wound quite slowly, moving forward one cell diameter (7 micrometers) an hour. It is known that they can move faster if the micro-environment is favorably modified. As was proved by Medawar, Bullogh and others, this movement can be speeded up by 3 p.c. using HPO at 2 ATA. This speeding up of the healing process can be easily understood by the fact that epidermal cells need oxygen for their migration and mitoses, and further that oxygen consumption of the epidermis rises with rising partial tension of oxygen. HPO of 2 ATA makes extra oxygen available to the moving cells both indirectly through the lungs and the systemic route to tissue fluids, and directly through the surface of the wound from outside.

The result of transplantation in burns depends in the main on the speed by which the transplant is taken, and consequently HPO appears to be even more useful. The good results attained by Perrins can be easily understood if we realize that oxygen is essential for metabolism of the healing wound for energy production, probably used in granulation tissue (in the main) for the production of ATP so essential for protein synthesis, stated by Hunt and Zederfelt (5). Molecular oxygen is further essential for the hydroxylation of protein in amino-acids which make up 25 p.c. of the links in the collagen molecule (Udenfriend). As stated by Ulkina (9), fibroblast will not proliferate in tissue cultures in the absence of oxygen; consequently epidermal regeneration and gain in tensile strength are delayed in animal experiments where wounds are exposed to reduced barometric pressure. Hull and others propose that the distance a given fibroblast can migrate from the nearest capillary is limited by the oxygen tension in the extracellular fluid. When the pO_2 is less than 10 mm Hg, the cells can no longer migrate, divide and synthetise collagen. The fibroblast near the capillary has a higher oxygen tension environment. As these cells produce collagen, new capillaries grow in and as each new capillary establishes a circulation, the supply of oxygen to the most distant cells is increased, they can now migrate and reproduce themselves. Thus, the rate at which the edges of the granulation tissue advance is limited by its blood supply. Administration of oxygen might accelerate the healing and revascularisation of the split skin graft; favourable results would explain, to a degree, the good effect of HPO therapy.

The well-known effect of the open treatment of burns seems to be multiplied by the application of HPO. Finally, we can state the bacterio-static effect of HPO against clostridial as well as other infections, and it therefore seems that Pseudomonas infection is treatable by using HPO. We can consequently state that HPO therapy speeds up the regeneration of tissue by bacteriostasis, and the healing of wounds with disturbed circulation.

On the basis of these findings we used HPO in retarded wound healing in so-called bed granulation tissue, when all routine methods failed. Further, we can prove that HPO speeded up the healing of donor sites, and made repeated grafting sooner possible. All of the 29 similar cases were influenced by HPO excellently.

In this chapter we may also deal with burns of bone and attending osteomyelitic complications. The influence of HPO was in these cases excellent, speeding up the healing and making it possible to take the grafts in a significantly short time. We applied this treatment in 5 patients.

Finally, we want to mention the last group of burned old and older patients where we used HPO. Patients over 50 years of age pose a specifically difficult chapter in the treatment of burns.

Of the many changes accompanying aging, those involving the cognitive function are the most striking. The processes involved in information storage, retrieval and conceptual efficiency are among those functions which are most affected by the changes associated with aging. Caird and Inglis (2) demonstrated a high correlation between age and short-term memory deficit. Hayes, Thompson and others proved that there exists a correlation between oxygen tension in the brain and the cognitive function. This was proved experimentally in induced cerebral circulatory arrest and effects of high altitude. This evidence leaves little doubt that growing oxygen tension in the brain may promote the cognitive function (Jacobs et al.). The saturation of the brain with oxygen depends on the brain blood flow, partial oxygen tension of the arterial blood and the intercapillary distance. It seems therefore possible that every condition which badly influences the mentioned circumstances may reduce the cognitive functions of the brain, short-term memory and conceptual efficiency. It is justified to believe that arteriosclerosis in the aged may lead to increased intercapillary distance and disturbed autoregulary mechanism of the cerebral capillary blood flow, and consequently to chronic hypoxia of the brain. Jacobs proved that increasing oxygen tension can refresh the brain functions. Our experience indicates that in patients suffering from chronic hypoxia who show very similar behavior and deficiency of brain, HPO treatment resulted in refreshing the brain function. In this case we treated not senile patients but patients with minor or gross limitations of the respiratory surface, or suffering from chronic intoxications.

In our four patients older than 60 years, HPO therapy was excellent. The patients became vivid, regained appetite, became more youthful, their expression and the quality of their hair changed, and the whole treatment was speeded up.

Concluding, we can state that HPO used in the 2nd stage of burn-disease (from the 3rd to 21st day) proved to be valuable in burns:

- with unstable granulating surfaces, resisting traditional methods (29 cases);
- of the bone and/or osteomyelitis (5 cases);
- of 60 years old and older patients (4 cases);

but did not prove to be valuable in burns:

- with already spread septicaemia (4 cases),
- with imperfect necrectomy (5 cases).

Summarising we state that HPO treatment is reasonable in both stages of the burns-disease, in selected groups of cases, which we recommend to you. We therefore state that HPO chambers are a very useful and important addition to the therapeutic tools securing and speeding up significantly the cure of the burned. On the basis of our experience we recommend HPO chambers to all departments dealing with burns.

References

1. Bullough. W. S. and Johnson, M. D. (1951): Epidermal mitotic activity and oxygen tension. Nature 167 : 488.
2. Caird, W. K. and Inglis, J. (1961): The short-term storage of auditori and visual two-channel digits by elderly patients with memory disorders. J. ment. Sci. 107 : 1067.
3. Inglis, J. and Caird, W. K. (1963): Age difference in successive responses to simultaneous stimulations. Canad. J. Psychol. 17 : 98.
4. Hayes, K. J. (1953): Anoxic and convulsive amnesia in rats. J. comp. physiol. Psychol. 46 : 216.
5. Hunt, T. K., Zederfelt, B. and Dunphy, J. E. (1967): Role of oxygen tension in healing. Surg. Ferum 18 : 3.
6. Medawar, P. B. (1948): The cultivation of mammalian adult skin epithelium. Quart. J. micr. Sci. 89 : 187.
7. Perrins, J. D. (1966): Hyperbaric oxygenation of ischemic skin flaps and pedicles. In: Hyperbaric Medicine. Eds. Brown and Cox, Nat. Acad. Sci. Nat. Res. Cncl. Washington.
8. Udenfriend, S. (1966): Formation of hydroxyproline in collagen. Science 152 : 1335.
9. Ulkina, O. T. (1964): Regeneration of the skin epithelium in healing wounds under normal conditions and at reduced atmospheric pressure. Biol. Abstr. 45 : 78585.
10. Thompson, R. (1957): The comparative effects of ECS and anoxia on memory. J. comp. physiol. Psychol. 50 : 379.

Š. Š., ZÚNZ — VSŽ,
044 53 Košice-Šaca, Czechoslovakia

ENTERAL TUBE FEEDING IN BURNED CHILDREN IN THE SHOCK AND TOXICOINFECTION PHASE

D. RANEV, L. MISHEVA and BL. SHINDARSKI

Emergency Medical Institute "Pirogov", Sofia, Bulgaria

In severely burned children, there develop catabolic processes with considerable protein decay in the shock and toxicoinfection phases. The necessary proteins cannot be supplied only parenterally, but additional enteral feeding is required.

In order to calculate the daily requirement of calories and nitrogen in burned patients, the body losses realized by exudation from the wound surfaces, the urine and the stool must be known (1, 4, 5, 8, 9).

The greatest nitrogen amounts are excreted in the urine. This is why it is in practice sufficient to safeguard balance between the nitrogen introduced into the organism and the nitrogen excreted in the urine in 24 hours, taking into consideration that the urea nitrogen represents 8/10 of the total nitrogen excreted with the urine (7).

The protein and calories needs in severe burns are considerable. According to various investigations they are 1–2.6 times higher in a burn case affecting 15 to 90 p.c. of the body surface than the basic metabolism requirements (2, 3).

The daily protein and calories needs are calculated for kg of body weight or for sq. m. body surface. According to Laurence and Angla de Soulier (6) it is difficult to establish a standard calorie diet in children — it must be an individual one. Wallace (11) proposes a diet containing proteins from 0.75 to 2 g/kg of body weight daily and 15 to 20 cal/kg

TABLE 1

Distribution of patients according to age and extent of burn

Age	Burn percentage			
	10–20 per cent	20–40 per cent	above 40 per cent	Total
1–3 years	2	7	2	11
3–7 years		6	1	7
7–14 years	2	2	1	5
Total	4	15	4	23

of body weight daily; Sutherland (10) gives 60 cal/kg of body weight daily + 1 g of proteins for every burn percentage. For the dosage of the calories and proteins the given quantities of blood and of its components need not be calculated. They are considered to be resources which can be consumed in the course of the burn. Depending on the surface damaged, the various authors propose various diets.

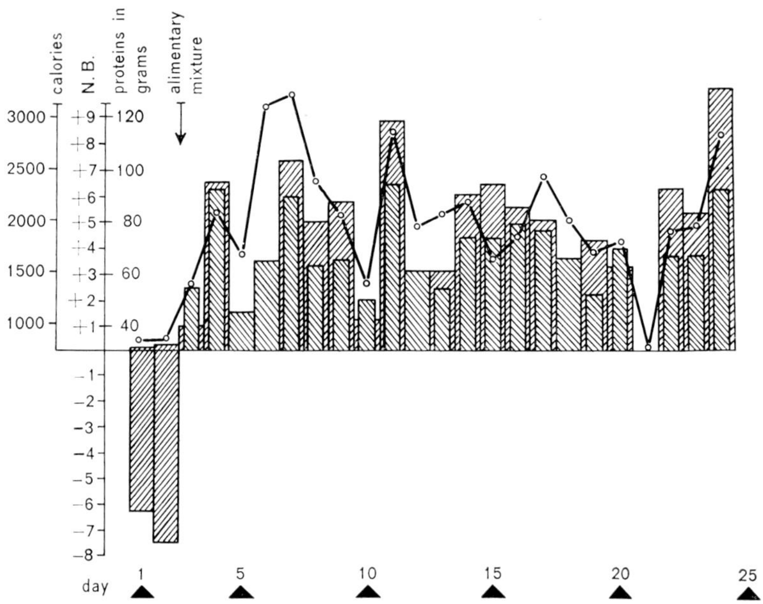

Fig. 1. Patient M. I. M., 7 years old, with 40 per cent burned surface area, degree IIIa-b. Case No. 10421/73 (▨ — nitrogen balance, ▧ — proteins taken orally, solid line — calories)

23 children from 1 to 14 years of age with 10 to 75 p.c. burns (3rd degree burns in over 5 p.c. of them) have been followed up (Table 1). The calories, fats and carbohydrates have been calculated every day, and twice a week (if necessary every day) the urea excreted in the 24-hours-diuresis has been investigated. On the grounds of these data we calculated the nitrogen balance according to the formula: nitrogen balance = all

TABLE 2

Required and taken amounts of food components

Age	Daily requirements				Taken — in 17 children			
	Protein	Fats	Carbo-hydrates	Calories	Protein	Fats	Carbo-hydrates	Calories
1–3 years	48–53	43–53	157	1330–1800	20–30	20–30	40–100	500–600
3–7 years	63–72	63–72	241	1880–1990	20–30	20–35	60–100	600–800
7–14 years	80–96	80–96	297–424	2380–3860	30–40	30–40	70–100	700–1200

TABLE 3

Products for the alimentary mixture

100 g product	Protein	Fats	Carbohydrates	Calories
Yoghurt from cow milk	3.8	4	2.5	63
Powder milk-Whole	28	28	31.5	504
Dried milk "Baby 1"	17	25	50	512
Dried milk "Vita-lact 2"	36	1	51	370
Humana 2	10	30	52	533
1 egg	6.1	5.5	0.4	77
Olive oil	0	99.9	0	883
Oil	0	99.9	0	883
Honey	0.5	0	78	322
Tomato juice	0.8	0.1	3.9	20
Lemon juice	0.5	0.2	8	25

proteins taken per os × 0.14 — the urea in the urine in g for 24 hours × 0.59. As the question of the calories required for the organism is comparatively well cleared up and their introduction is more accessible, we take into consideration the physiological daily needs of the children when prescribing them.

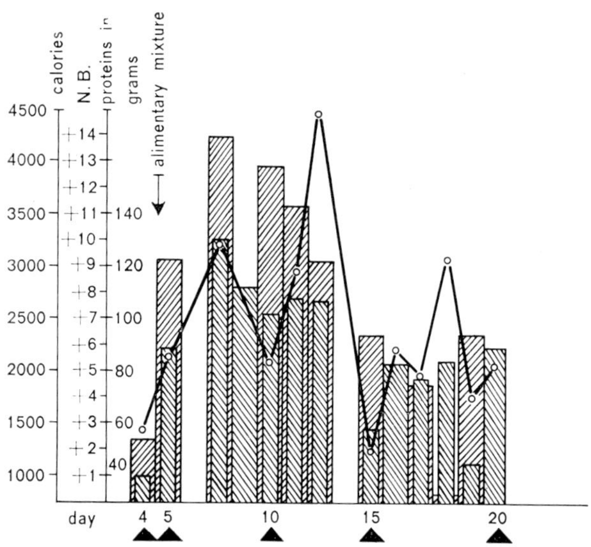

Fig. 2. Patient T. I. H., 5 years old, with 40 per cent burned surface area, degree IIIa–b. Case No. 7839/73 (see also legends to Fig. 1)

Shock phase. As the children take only water during the first two days after the burn, in fractions of 10–20 ml p/h, the nitrogen balance is negative. On the third day when they begin to take thin food (yoghurt or milk, stewed fruit, jelly, etc.), the nitrogen balance becomes slightly positive (Fig. 1).

Toxicoinfection phase. In this stage the patients are given mechanically well prepared and chemically sparing food. In spite of this, the children take rather less than are the daily needs (Table 2). In view of this, we applied additional tube feeding with alimentary mixture in 23 children treated in the burned children department of the Clinic for Burns and Plastic Surgery. The alimentary mixture was prepared with the products given in Table 3 and water or milk. It must be watery and pass freely through the tube.

Indications for tube feeding: 1. In anorexia or when the children are not able to take necessary proteins and calories. The tube makes it possible to give fractioned alimentary mixture by the drop system day and night. Additional alimentation is given mainly in the night hours, when the children are asleep so that they might take the diet prescribed in the day.

2. In tracheostomy or intubation in airways burns or in respiratory insufficiency due to circulatory or inflammatory changes.

3. In deep face or mouth burns which do not permit the child to eat.

4. Bandage after operation of deep face burns.

Quality of the alimentary mixture: a) The calories given with the alimentary mixture must supplement the daily needs (and the child tolerates well the feeding) to exceed these by 20 to 40 per cent. b) Proteins are given to supplement those taken orally until a positive nitrogen balance is obtained — +5 to +7, and in older children to +10 — +12.

c) The water or the milk in the alimentary mixture is from 400 to 600 ml. The remaining water amount necessary for the daily requirement is taken separately per os. d) Vitamins — vit. "C", 2 ampules and vitamins: "B_1" and "B_6" 1 amp. daily, e) Potassium — 2 mE/kg weight, and in case of hypopotassaemia to 4 mE/kg/weight daily, bicarbonate of sodium — in local treatment with acidizing solutions and Sulfamylon.

The *quantity of the alimentary mixture* for children reaches a maximum value of 600 to 800 ml. and is divided in 4–5 portions, each of them from 50 to 150 ml.

Rhythm of the alimentation: The night hours proved to be most convenient, when the child is asleep and can take the additional feeding in drops; it is given at 20, 23, 2 and 5 o'clock.

Tolerance of the alimentary mixture is good. Vomiting and intolerence of the tube have been observed in two children, where the tube feeding was stopped.

All children followed up recovered.

Conclusions

In children with severe burns, there develop catabolic processes with considerable protein decay in the shock and toxicoinfection phases. The necessary proteins cannot be supplied only parenterally, which requires additional enteral feeding. The follow-up of 23 children, aged 1 to 14 years, with 10 to 75 per cent burns (3rd degree above 5 p.c.), showed that in the shock and toxicoinfection phases the patients take per os calories and proteins far under the daily needs. This leads to a negative nitrogen balance which is calculated on the basis of the proteins taken and the urea excreted with the urine.

Supplementary feeding with an alimentary mixture rich in proteins and calories introduced by tube, makes the nitrogen balance positive and greatly improves the course and the issue of the disease.

References

1. Artz, G. P. and Moncrief, J. A. (1967): The Treatment of Burns, 2nd Ed. Philadelphia, W. B. Saunders Company.
2. Cope, O., Hardi, G. L., Quijano, L., Rovit, R. L., Stanbury, J. B. and Wight, A. (1953): Metabolic rate and thyroid function following acute thermal trauma in man. Ann. Surg. 137 : 165.
3. Harrison, H. N., Moncrief, J. A., Duckett, F. W. and Mason, A. D. (1964): The relation-

ship between energy metabolism and water loss from vaporization in severely burned patients. Surgery 56 : 203.
4. Henry, R. I. (1966): Clinical Chemistry. Principles and Techniques. New York, Harper and Row.
5. Kayser, J. M. (1948): Metabolic study of burn cases. Ann. Surg. 127 : 605.
6. Laurence, G. et Angla de Saulier, (1958): 482 cas de brûlés chez l'enfant. Mém. Acad. Chir. 84 : 820.
7. Loirat, Ph. (1970): L'alimentation parentérale exclusive et prolongée. Thèse Faculté de Médecine de Paris.
8. Nylen, B. and Wallenius, G. (1961): The protein loss via exudation from burns and granulating wound surfaces. Acta chir. scand. 122 : 97.
9. Reiss, E., Pearson, E. and Arzt, C. P. (1956): The metabolic response to burns. J. clin. Invest. 35 : 62.
10. Sutherland, A. B. and Batchelor, A. D. K. (1966): Nitrogen balance in burned children. In: Research in Burns, Livingstone, Edinburgh, 147.
11. Wallace, A. B. (1958): Present outlook on burns. Plast. reconstr. Surg. 21 : 243.

D. R., Emergency Medical Inst.
„Pirogov“,
Sofia, Bulgaria

CRITERIA, PRINCIPLES AND RESULTS OF THE TREATMENT OF BURN DISEASE

A. A. SHALIMOV, F. P. VOROBYEV, D. E. PEKARSKII
and T. G. GRIGOREVA

Burns Centre, Research Institute of General and Emergency Surgery, Kharkov, USSR

Everyday clinical practice shows that disturbances of homoeostasis in burn victims depend not only on the severity of the lesion, but also on additional factors, which have been studied but not yet fully elucidated. Contemporary clinical practice is not, therefore, any more content with the etiological, anatomical, and even clinical diagnoses of burns.

Clinicians have been feeling the need of a pathophysiological diagnosis in burn victims, because the disturbances of the physiological balance in the patients' organisms vary to such an extent that a reliable symptomatic reparation of the disturbances is hardly possible and feasible, and sometimes would not even serve any rational purpose.

Our experience gained in the treatment of 5677 patients with burns between 1966 1972 shows that the efforts made to establish a pathophysiological diagnosis are reflected in favourable therapeutic results, because such a diagnosis helps adapt the treatment to individual requirements aimed at restitution of the disturbed homoeostasis. This is the specific feature of our organizational and therapeutic tactics.

In our concept, burn shock has to be considered not a complication of the injury, but a regular response of the organism to the trauma and, moreover, an inevitable stage of the burn disease. From the pathophysiological point of view, however, the burn shock is a dynamic process involving increasing insufficiency of the central, regional and peripheral circulation as well as changes in the rheological properties of blood. Haemodynamic disturbances elicit disturbances in and functional weakening of a variety of organs and systems, with resulting disorders in a variety of metabolic processes.

The diagnosis of burn shock therefore requires speedy checking of the basic haemodynamic indicators in burn victims. Findings of changes in the absolute values of haemodynamic indicators, and the existence of characteristic combinations of such changes, allowed us to identify burn shock in 444 patients, that is 7.8 per cent of the total number of burn victims treated.

Being a pathological process passing through successive phases, burn shock proceeds in a way in which a very great variety of nonspecific factors and adaptive reactions take turn in joining the pathophysiological mechanism. Consequently, the clinical presentation of burn shock depends on the severity of the thermal lesion as well as on the patient's adaptive and compensatory reactions.

Clinical experience shows that in a preponderant majority of burn victims the course of burn shock passes through the following three consecutive phases: (1) the compensation phase, lasting 4–6 hours after the accident; (2) the decompensation phase, extending between the 7th and 24th hours; and (3) the stabilization phase, extending between the 25th and 48th hours after the accident. The organizational and therapeutic problems involved in the individual phases of shock development are considerably different. In the first stage, i.e. in the compensation phase of shock the patients tolerate transport to a specialized hospital very well. Leaving aside the question whether transport is always mandatory, we feel justified to state on the basis of our experiences with more than 170 patients that patients in the first phase of shock are fit for transport.

In our search for as reliable criteria as possible for the appraisal of the state of a patient in shock, we analyzed several comprehensive indicators reflecting the vascular tone level, oxygen turnover and oxygen uptake level in tissues disturbed in consequence of shock. Accepting the total peripheral vascular resistance as a function of the systemic circulation, we measured the patients' vascular tone in the course of all of the phases of burn shock (Table 1).

TABLE 1

Vascular tone in patients in state of burn shock

	Phase of shock		
	1st	2nd	3rd
$\frac{\text{dyn.sec.cm}^{-5}}{\text{l/min.m}^2}$	521.5 ± 43.4	290.2 ± 20.7	418.0 ± 32.1

The data presented in Table 1 confirm the general trend of haemodynamic disturbances in burn shock: the vascular tone rises in the first phase, sinks in the second phase and stabilizes in the third phase of shock. The data not only inform about the changes occurring in the factors participating in the formation of the vascular tone, but also point to the necessity to use such therapeutic means for burn shock which effectively influence the vascular tone as well as the entire circulation.

An analysis of the oxygen turnover in patients with burn shock offered a general picture of the functions of external respiration (oxygen uptake), haemodynamics (oxygen transport), and metabolism (oxygen utilization), and thus made possible an assessment of the overall state of external and internal tissue respiration in the organism.

The following indicators of oxygen turnover were investigated:

1. Effective transport of oxygen, that is, the capacity of oxygen extraction per liter of cardiac output;
2. Index of relative peripheral blood shunt, reflecting the existence and function of pathological arteriovenous shunts — the ratio between peripheral vascular resistance and the effective transport of oxygen;
3. Coefficient of oxygen utilization;
4. Intensity of anaerobic metabolism.

The last two indicators make it possible to appraise the degree of oxygen utilization in metabolic processes.

The above indicators of oxygen turnover were also checked in all phases of burn shock (Table 2).

From this table, the phasic character of the course of burn shock is also evident. Thus,

TABLE 2

Oxygen turnover in patients with burn shock

Indicators	Phase of shock		
	1st	2nd	3rd
EOT $\frac{ml}{l/min.m^2}$	68.6 ± 4.6	127.8 ± 7.9	38.3 ± 2.7
RPS $\frac{dyn.sec.cm^{-5}}{ml/l.min.m^2}$	26.1 ± 2.4	12.1 ± 1.0	54.8 ± 4.2
COU (in per cent)	36.8 ± 4.6	8.6 ± 0.9	29.9 ± 2.7
IAM (in per cent)	37.6 ± 2.7	76.1 ± 5.8	10.7 ± 0.9

EOT — effective oxygen transport
RPS — index of relative peripheral shunt
COU — coefficient of oxygen utilization
IAM — coefficient of intensity of anaerobic metabolism

for example, in the second — decompensation — phase of the shock the oxygen utilization steeply falls; consequently, the intensity of anaerobic metabolism increases, although effective oxygen transport increases and the index of relative peripheral blood shunt decreases.

In view of the high informative value of data on oxygen turnover for the assessment of the patient's condition, we attempted to find a single indicator expressing the ratio between aerobic and anaerobic processes and simultaneously serviceable as a prognostic criterion in burn victims. Such an indicator was found in the excess lactate level in mixed venous blood.

The excess lactate level in mixed venous blood was estimated in 108 patients with burns varying in severity and extent during the first days after the accident. The data obtained are presented in Table 3.

TABLE 3

Excess lactate levels (in meq/liter) in state of burn shock

Frank's coefficient	Excess lactate level
up to 30	1.03 ± 0.05
31–60	1.49 ± 0.12
61–90	2.32 ± 0.17
91–120	3.44 ± 0.32
over 120	3.97 ± 0.38

The table shows that along with increasing severity of the thermal injury, that is, with increasing deterioration of the blood supply to tissues, the excess lactate level rises in patients with burn shock.

To elucidate how far the excess lactate level is usable as an indicator of reversibility of burn shock and of the prognosis of the latter's course, we compared the levels found in three groups of patients (Table 4).

TABLE 4

Excess lactate levels in patients with different outcomes of burn disease

Group of patients those who	Excess lactate level	Statistical significance	
		P_1	P_2
died in state of burn shock	4.49 ± 0.51		
recovered from shock, but died in subsequent stages of burn disease	2.98 ± 0.32	< 0.02	
healed	1.46 ± 0.16	< 0.001	< 0.01

The results showed that the excess lactate level in mixed venous blood not only reflects the severity of the condition of a patient with thermal lesion, but may also serve as a reliable prognostic criterion in burn shock. In the light of our findings, an excess lactate level higher than 2 meq/liter indicates a poor prognosis, and a level higher than 4 meq/liter, an infaust prognosis.

Consequently, investigations of the oxygen turnover and the ratio between aerobic and anaerobic metabolic processes in patients with burn shock helped find a reliable prognostic criterion in the burn disease, in the form of the excess lactate level in the patient's mixed venous blood.

As confirmed by extensive investigations, changes in basic haemodynamic indicators in burn victims are dependent primarily on the severity of the thermal lesion, in particular on the magnitude of the area of deep burn, and on the length of time elapsed since the accident. Besides, there exist mutual interactions and certain mutual relationships among individual basic haemodynamic indicators.

Thus, for example, a direct linear correlation was found to exist between the circulating blood volume and the cardiac stroke volume in burn shock. We considered it important, however, to quantify the closeness of the correlation between the above indicators, differentiated with respect to the severity of the thermal lesion as well as to the length of time elapsed since the accident.

In patients with skin destroyed on less than 10 per cent of body surface, the deviations of the values of circulating blood volume from the control values were statistically insignificant ($p > 0.5$; 0.2; 0.5). The search for correlations between the circulating blood volume and the cardiac stroke volume in these patients showed that the coefficient of correlation between both indicators was 0.31 ± 0.22 ($P > 0.1$), attesting to a very poor correlation. A certain decrease in the systolic blood volume in the first stage of burn disease with no great extent of thermal lesions, is therefore, unconnected with changes in the circulating blood volume.

In patients with burns of major severity, the closeness of the correlation between the cardiac stroke volume and the circulating blood volume is dependent on the development phase of burn shock (Tab. 5).

The data in this table convincingly document that in patients with deep burns on more than 10 per cent of body surface, the decrease in the stroke volume seen in the first two phases of burn shock does not essentially result from decreased venous return. The decrease in the stroke volume is evidently ascribable to some other causes (toxic, intracardiac, and others). In the further course of burn shock, however, hypovolaemia becomes

TABLE 5

Correlation coefficients between stroke index and circulating blood volume in patients with burns in various phases of shock

Indicator	Normal values	Phase of shock		
		1st	2nd	3rd
	A — Loss of skin on 11–20 per cent of body surface			
Stroke index ml/m²	41.4 ± 4.1	29.0 ± 4.24 < 0.001	27.9 ± 5.05 < 0.001	30.6 ± 3.7 < 0.001
Circulating blood volume ml/kg	70.3 ± 7.3	48.2 ± 10.2 < 0.001	49.4 ± 9.2 < 0.001	57.5 ± 10.7 < 0.001
Coefficient of correlation		0.42 ± 0.22 > 0.1	0.47 ± 0.2 > 0.1	0.85 ± 0.07 < 0.001
	B — Loss of skin on more than 20 per cent of body surface			
Stroke index ml/m²	41.4 ± 4.1	25.2 ± 1.93 < 0.001	24.4 ± 3.18 < 0.001	26.6 ± 2.3 < 0.001
Circulating blood volume ml/kg	70.3 ± 7.3	72.0 ± 3.1 > 0.5	43.4 ± 6.7 < 0.02	55.4 ± 6.5 < 0.01
Coefficient of correlation		0.28 ± 0.24 > 0.1	0.23 ± 0.26 > 0.1	0.95 ± 0.04 < 0.001

the prime factor responsible for insufficient cardiac performance. In the third phase of burn shock, the magnitudes of the correlation coefficients testify to very close correlations between the circulating blood volume and the cardiac stroke volume: 0.85 ± 0.07 and 0.95 ± 0.04. On the day following after a thermal lesion which had led to a loss of skin on more than 10 per cent of body surface, the decrease in cardiac performance is therefore primarily due to a decrease in the circulating blood volume. These findings must not be evidently disregarded in the choice of rational and efficient antishock treatment.

The magnitudes of cardiac performance and peripheral vascular resistance exhibit a hyperbolic correlation. Cardiac performance increases if peripheral vascular resistance decreases.

The mathematical dependence between the cardiac index and peripheral vascular resistance in patients with burns was calculated on the basis of our clinical material, and expressed by the formula

$$CI = 230 \times PVR^{-0.06},$$

where CI — cardiac index; PVR — peripheral vascular resistance; 230 and 0.06 — constants.

The validity of this dependence was confirmed by calculations of the cardiac index in control subjects, using the actual values of peripheral vascular resistance and the above formula.

Consequently, a decrease in peripheral vascular resistance is associated with an increase in the cardiac output. On the basis of this finding, when treating burn shock, we performed blockade of the adrenergic systems; our experiences with this blockade involve more than 135 patients with burn shock treated at our clinic.

The favourable effect of adrenolytic agents on the haemodynamics in patients in the state of burn shock consists primarily in a substantial reduction of the peripheral vascular resistance and, in consequence, also increases in the cardiac output and cardiac stroke volume. There results, as a rule, a stabilization of haemodynamics in the burn victims.

Apart from the haemodynamic effect common for all adrenolytic agents, the individual preparations in this group exhibit certain additional specific activities: neuroleptics produce neurovegetative sedation, ganglion blockers help in counteracting respiratory insufficiency and heart failure, antiadrenergic agents remove tachycardia, and alpha-adrenergic receptor blockers considerably modify the entire circulation.

Finally, a follow-up analysis of the haemodynamic indicators in the course of burn shock and of their typical clinical manifestations, respecting their dependence on the phase of the shock, made possible a definition of indications for a differentiated administration of pharmacotherapeutic agents actively influencing the vascular tone in a wide variety of blood circulation disturbances and other clinical symptoms of burn shock.

In the first phase of burn shock, we consider the following agents to be indicated:

1. neuroleptics;
2. ganglion blocking agents, making use of tachyphylactic resistance to their hypotensive action;
3. sympatholytics;
4. alpha-adrenergic receptor blockers.

In the second phase of burn shock, ganglion blockade may be used by concurrent administration of ganglion blocking agents and sympathomimetics.

Differentiated indications of adrenolytic therapy in burn shock

1st phase of shock

General indication	General counter-indication
Attainment of high-degree sympathetic nervous tone	Arterial hypotension

Neuroleptics

Clinical indications:

1. psychomotor agitation
2. aggregated thermal lesions
3. period before start of hospital treatment
4. postponement of start, and restriction of intensity of antishock treatment

Ganglion blockade on the basis of tachyphylaxis

Clinical indications:

1. disturbances in lesser circulation with respiratory difficulties; heart failure
2. heart insufficiency;
3. portal hypertension.

Sympatholytics

Clinical indications:

haemodynamic disturbances
accompanied by tachycardia

alpha-Adrenergic receptor blockade

Clinical indications:

disturbances of entire circulation
persisting over several hours
despite antishock treatment

2nd phase of shock

Ganglion blockade by concurrent administration of ganglion blockers and sympathomimetics

Clinical indications:

pathological fluid cumulation
in consequence of vasoplegia

It has to be noted that the differentiated indications of adrenergic blocking therapy of burn shock are based on extensive clinical experience. In all patients in whom adrenergic system blockade was performed, convincing clinical effects and a considerable improvement in the blood circulation were achieved. No complications were observed.

The use of adrenergic receptor blockers, although not yet usual in the treatment of burn shock, leads, in the light of our experiences, to a considerable improvement in the circulation and facilitates the rehabilitation of the patients. Attention is again drawn to the importance of a differentiation of indications, the definition of the suitability, conditions and possibilities of administrating neuroleptics, ganglion blockers, sympatholytics and adrenergic receptor blockers in the treatment of burn shock. Our results help to make more effective and more purposeful use of agents regulating the vascular tone in comprehensive care aimed at resuscitation of burn victims.

Regulation of the blood circulation is, in our opinion, of cardinal importance in the treatment of burn shock. Its usefulness has been proved in more than 90 per cent of the patients admitted to our clinic with manifest burn shock syndrome. Furthermore, earliest possible stabilization of the state of the afflicted patients makes possible surgical treatment aimed at repairing the skin destroyed by burns already at the early stage of the lesion. The total death rate of patients operated upon was about 11 per cent at our clinic.

D. E. P., Balakireva 1,
310018 Kharkov, USSR

SEPTICAEMIA

CONTEMPORARY PROBLEMS OF INFECTION IN BURNS

L. PÁVKOVÁ and Z. KONÍČKOVÁ

Laboratory of Plastic Surgery, Czechoslovak Academy of Sciences, Prague, and Burns Centre, Faculty of Hygiene, Charles University, Prague, Czechoslovakia

Though the treatment of burns has undergone great development due to a more profound knowledge of the possibilities to influence the course of metabolic processes, the problem of infection still remains unsolved. In burns, infection contributes markedly to the mortality rate, slows down the healing process and elevates the cost of treatment.

Bacterial contamination of the burn wound cannot be totally avoided. In many stations, though, the character of infection and its damaging influence vary. According to Lowbury, the development of nosocomial infection is in a direct relation to the overall number of burns treated in the unit, to the proportion of extensive burns and to the proportion of patients transferred from other hospitals; infection is in an indirect relation to the number of hospital personnel and to the possibilities of patients isolation. The development of infection may be also influenced by different methods of treatment used in various hospitals.

The high susceptibility of burned patients to infection is well known. This may be caused by several factors, the most important of which is doubtless the loss of natural barrier represented by skin. Microcirculatory changes developing in the vicinity of thermally damaged tissue represent also an important factor, as they are preventing the access of leukocytes to the injured area. Phagocytic capacity of leukocytes remains unchanged, but their capacity to kill bacteria they have devoured, decreases.

We do not have as yet sufficient knowledge of the changes in the antibody production. In recent years, the changes of immunoglobulins were studied, but the results of different studies vary. A clear relation between the changes in immunoglobulin levels and between the development of infection and the grave general state of the patient could not be defined so far.

Nevertheless a clear relation can be defined between the course of the burn illness and the RES function, which appears to be of prominent importance in the arsenal of the defences of a burned organism.

In burned patients, the capacity of RES is being overburdened the RES having to dispose of catabolic products, necrotic tissues and bacterial toxins, phagocyted and free microbes. This may result in an accumulation of non-toxic products, which in an abnormal quantity can have a toxic effect.

Therefore, during the treatment of the burn illness, all the therapy that might additionally burden the RES, should be avoided such as certain antibiotics, HMW dextran, halothane, etc. A deep metabolic disharmony developing in all severe burns influences bacterial invasion and is in turn influenced by infection strongly, thus completing a vicious circle.

As it appears, antibiotics did neither solve nor simplify the problem of burn infection. Indiscriminate use of antibiotics lowered the general resistance of population; it also disturbed microbial patterns in human organism, favouring resistant microbes. It is important to stress that we are now encountering dangerous "potential pathogens" that in the past used to be harmless. This fact may be best illustrated by the changes in burn wound microbial patterns observed during the last 20 years in the Prague Center.

It is a common experience in many burns stations that Streptococcus haemolyticus, which used to be predominant, is now rare. Staphylococcus aureus, which predominated in later years, still has a high frequency, but its pathogenic effect is now of secondary importance. At present, the highest importance may be attributed to Pseudomonas aeruginosa. According to recent literature, though, a new danger is represented by the appearance of fungi in burn wound. A possibility of virus infection also has to be taken into consideration.

Staphylococcus aureus still represents an unpleasant complication of local healing in the later stages of the burn illness. It may be of interest that in several cases local Staphylococcus aureus infection was successfully combatted in the Prague Burns Centre by fagotherapy.

Generalized infection, mainly in its chronic form, represents the greatest problem in the treatment of extensive burns. During septicaemia, the burn wound microbial pattern of an individual patient is constantly changing; this is specific for burns and is rarely encountered in other surgical infection. It may be presumed that manifestations of long-lasting septicaemia are often induced by endotoxaemia as such.

In the treatment of infection, a combination of therapeutical measure must be applied. Surgical procedures, necrectomy and transplantation are still of utmost importance. Local bacteriostatic therapy is certainly of considerable value, but it cannot always prevent generalized infection. An indispensable primary therapeutical factor is the care for the general state of the patient and his energetic and metabolic balance.

As antibiotics apparently cannot completely solve the problem of infection, other means of combatting bacteria must be searched for. More interest should now be devoted to specific immunotherapy, both passive and active. (It is quite possible that the favourable results we met with after convalescent sera application may have been due to passive immunisation of the patients treated.) Nevertheless, non-specific defences of the organism which have long been neglected, or even supressed, deserve further study as well.

Yet it is not likely that immunotherapy only will suffice in the treatment of burn infection. Generalized infection in extensive burns represents a complex problem requiring complex therapy adapted dynamically to laboratory results and individual situation. The greater the arsenal of preventive diagnostic and therapeutical tools, the better will be the results.

Therefore, we should like to thank all speakers in this section who by their contribution will further our knowledge of what seems to be the key problem of the burn illness.

L. P., Legerova 63,
120 00 Praha 2, Czechoslovakia

CONTAMINATION OF BURN WOUND IN PRAGUE BURNS CENTER IN 1969–1972

T. PELLAR, L. PÁVKOVÁ, and R. KÖNIGOVÁ

Institute of Microbiology, Faculty of Hygiene, Prague Laboratory of Plastic Surgery, Academy of Sciences and Burns Center, University Hospital, Prague, Czechoslovakia

Our study demonstrates the bacteriological contamination (Table 1) of the burned surface of patients admitted between January 1969 and December 1972. The material was examined in the same laboratory using the same methods. The total number of bacteriological swabs was 4006. Ten per cent of the examined samples were negative every year. The microbes most frequently isolated were Staphylococcus aureus, Pseudomonas aeruginosa, Proteus, Streptococci haemolyt., Escherichia coli. The other microbes were found in less than 2.5 per cent on the burned area surface (per year) (Table 2).

TABLE 1

The total number of positive bacteriological examinations throughout the years 1969–1972

Years	Number of swabs
1969	666
1970	851
1971	1 347
1972	1 142
Total	4 006

Staphylo aureus was isolated approximately in 75 per cent of all bacteriological findings. Table 2 points out the decrease of Streptococci haemolyt. from 20.5 per cent in 1969 to only 5.2 per cent in 1972. In the past years, this microbe used to be the threat in all exposed wounds.

Table 3 shows the relation between the microbes occurring as monoculture and those appearing in mixed infections. The most frequent agent isolated from burn wound was Staphylo aureus — more than 50 per cent. Pseudomonas aerug. was found in 25 per cent and Strepto haemol. in 20 per cent. The rare occurrence of Escherichia coli and Proteus in monoculture is a proof that those microbes feature the secondary contamination.

TABLE 2

The microbes most frequently isolated on burned surfaces in 1969–1972, in absolute numbers and in percentage of all positive examinations

Microbe	1969		1970		1971		1972		Total	
	A	per cent	A	per cent	A	per cent	A	per cent	A	per cent
St. aureus	532	79.8	674	79.2	939	69.7	803	70.3	2948	73.6
Ps. aerugin.	136	20.4	163	19.1	256	19.0	289	25.3	844	21.1
Proteus	148	22.2	176	20.1	136	10.1	111	9.7	571	14.3
Esch. coli	34	5.1	96	11.3	132	9.8	124	10.9	386	9.6
Str. haemol.	137	20.5	66	7.7	93	6.9	59	5.2	355	8.9

TABLE 3

Percentage of microbes isolated in monoculture of the total number of microbes on burned surfaces

Microbe	1969		1970		1971		1972		Total	
	A	per cent	A	per cent	A	per cent	A	per cent	A	per cent
St. aureus	218	40.9	334	49.8	487	51.8	469	58.4	1508	51.3
Ps. aerugin.	22	16.2	16	9.8	89	34.8	96	33.2	223	26.4
Str. haemol.	23	16.8	14	21.2	24	25.8	12	20.3	73	20.6
Proteus	18	12.1	43	24.4	15	11.0	18	16.2	94	16.6
Esch. coli	1		10	10.4	18	13.6	33	26.6	62	16.1

TABLE 4

Combinations of various types of microbes isolated on burned sufaces

Bacterial colonization	1969–1972	Per cent
St. aureus + Ps. aeruginosa	332	8.3
St. aureus + Proteus	236	5.9
St. aureus + Str. haemolyticus	206	5.0
St. aureus + Esch. coli	80	2.0
Ps. auruginosa + Proteus	54	1.4
St. aureus + Ps. aeruginosa + Proteus	61	1.5

Table 4 illustrates the usual combinations of microbes throughout the last years. Recently, we have repeatedly observed gram-negative threads which do not pertain either to the Enterobacteriaceae or to Pseudomonadales. We have classified, provisionally this microbe to the family of Achromobacter according to its biochemical properties. Its significance regarding the course and prognosis of burn illness is not yet quite clear. On the other hand, its presence on the burned surface must not be neglected.

The cross infection studies have been carried out in many Burns Units and discussions on so-called hospital strains continue. Certain strains are more resistant to inimical conditions and also better adapted to the given hospital environment, hence the emergence of resident strains. The sensitivity to antibiotics is very low, often only one of the highest antibiotics is found to be effective (*in vitro*).

With respect to the studies of other authors dealing with the determinations and occurrence of Staphylo aureus and Pseudomonas aerug. in burn wound, we draw attention to the third most frequent microbe in extensive burns — Proteus. We have classified Proteus not only biochemically, but also we have carried out the serological identification. Specific O-antigen has been determined by means of homologous hyperimmune rabbit antiserum in more than 150 strains. Thus, we have specified more than 30 different serological groups. This high dispersion of strains is contradictory to the hypothesis of hospital strains. We have also been finding various serotypes of Proteus in one patient throughout his staying in the ward.

Kotasová has communicated similar results in her work dealing with Pseudomonas aeruginosa.

In extensive burns we cannot be satisfied with only qualitative examinations of microbes in burn wound. In the complicated cases it is indispensible to know more about the count of different microbes present on the searched surface.

We have been using several semiquantitative methods: print on microscopic glass or transfer by means of filtering paper. Finally, we have tried the method well known in other specialities, i.e. print method by means of Duchoslav plate, which is a shallow plate filled with blood agar. Its surface is hemispherical bulging above the edge of the plate. The whole surface (10 square centimeters) takes the print. The used blood agar guarantees the growth of all microbes usually contaminating the burn wound. The colonies can be counted accurately up to 300 and approximately up to 1000 colonies. At the same time, we take swabs from the same spot, first for checking, secondly, for easier and briefer detection of the sensitivity to antibiotics.

The clinical use of this method is the subject of the next paper.

T. P., Institute of Microbiology,
Šrobárova 50,
100 34 Praha 10, Czechoslovakia

BACTERIOLOGICAL EXAMINATION OF BURN WOUNDS BY MEANS OF SEMIQUANTITATIVE METHOD

L. PÁVKOVÁ, T. PELLAR, R. KÖNIGOVÁ, V. VACEK and R. VRABEC

Laboratory of Plastic Surgery, Academy of Sciences, Department of Microbiology, Faculty of Hygiene, Burns Center, Faculty of Hygiene, Charles University, Prague, Czechoslovakia

In the last two years, we have examined bacterial wound contamination in our severely burned patients by means of the semiquantitative method.

A series of 62 severely burned patiens treated in the intensive care ward of Burns Center in Prague, were tested by this method. Burned areas involved more than 20 per cent of the total body surface. The semiquantitative examination of the wound infection

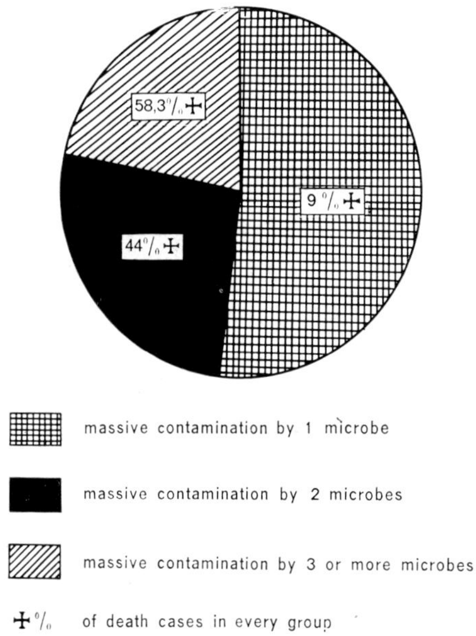

Fig. 1. Pure and mixed bacterial culture isolated from the burn wound.

TABLE 1

Microbes isolated from the burn wound in 62 severely burned patients

Monoculture

Microbes	No of cases	Per cent
staph. aureus	15	24.2
ps. aeruginosa	16	25.8
achromobacter	1	1.6

Mixed culture two microbes

Microbes	No of cases	Per cent
ps. aeruginosa + staph. aureus	11	17.7
ps. aeruginosa + proteus	4	6.45
ps. aeruginosa + achromobacter	1	1.6
staph. aureus + proteus	1	1.6
staph. aureus + achromobacter	1	1.6

Three and more microbes

	No of cases	Per cent
ps. aeruginosa + staph. aureus + achromobacter	2	3.2
ps. aeruginosa + staph. aureus + proteus	3	4.8
ps. aeruginosa + achromobacter + e. coli	3	4.8
proteus + e. coli + achromobacter	1	1.6
staph. aureus + enterobacter + achromobacter	2	3.2
ps. aeruginosa + proteus + staph. aureus + achromobacter	1	1.6

was perfomed twice a week during the course of the burn illness. At the same time the antibiogram was being determined.

Table 1 gives the survey of microbes which were cultivated from the burn wound. The table has been divided into three parts according to the number of bacterial strains found on burned surfaces. Cases in which one microbial strain was isolated in high numbers from the beginning to the end of the burn illness, were designated as mono-culture, because the other microbes, if present, were found in very low counts and appeared only occasionally. In cases, where two or more microbes were growing together in approximately identical concentration during a longer period, the findings were qualified as mixed infection. The frequency of microbes after cultivation was characterised by the number of colonies of microbes. Cases with innumerable and confluent colonies were designated as massive infection.

Fig. 1 shows the relation between mixed infection and monocultures. In our group of patients there appeared 51 per cent of monocultures. The frequency of Staphylococcus aureus was equal to the occurrence of Pseudomonas aeruginosa. Achromobacter was isolated only in one case. Two different microbes contaminated 29 per cent of cases and three microbes — 20 per cent. The fatalities were in reversed relation. Majority of deaths was noticed in the last group, where the extensive burned surface was massively contaminated by three different microbes during the whole period of treatment.

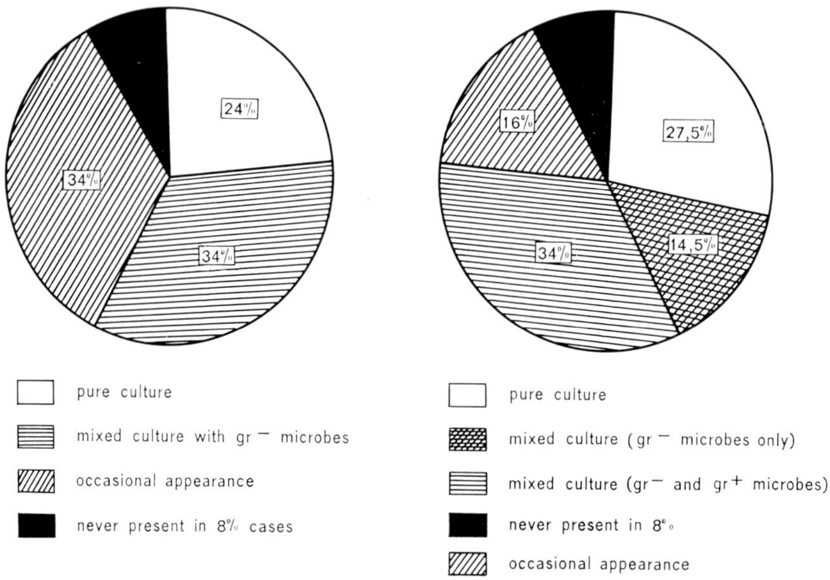

Fig. 2. Left: Appearance of Staphylococcus aureus in burn wound. Right: Appearance of gram-negati ve microbes in burn wound.

Fig. 2 demonstrates the fact that the gram-negative infection was far more frequent (42 per cent) than contamination by gram-positive microbes (24 per cent only). Gram-positive infection in our cases was represented by Staphylococcus aureus. Staphylococcus aureus in mono-culture was mostly discovered in minor burns and only exceptionally was it the cause of infection with general manifestation. On the contrary its presence in mixed culture with massive growth of gram-negatives is considered to be very serious.

Achromobacter, gram-negative thread, forms a special group. This microbe was brought to the Intensive Care Ward by one of severely burned patients, transferred from a county hospital about one year ago. Since then, this microbe has appeared on extensive deep burns in other patients. Its sensitivity to antibiotics is very low and the strains sensitive only to Polymyxin are not rare.

Fig 3 shows its occurrence in our group. It is not without interest that 7 patiensts out of 10, with massive contamination by this microbe, died. It is difficult to say what role this microbe was playing regarding the cause of death. In the future, we certainly should like to study the identity of this microbe and its conditional pathogenity.

In conclusion, we should like to recommend the semiquantitative method for clinical use. In cases of mixed infection with negative hemocultures the semiquantitative method enables the physician to detect the microbe which may be responsible for the serious condition of the patient and thus it also helps the physician to choose the right therapeutical measures to combat this microbe.

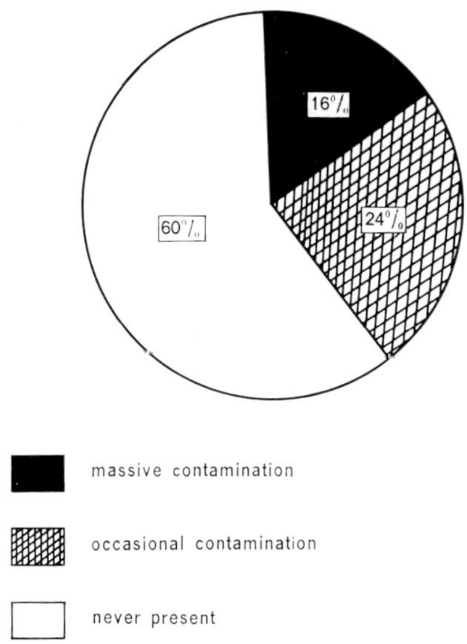

Fig. 3. Appearance of Achromobacter in the burn wound.

REFERENCES

1. McNAUGHT, W. (1971): Bacteriological monitoring of burns using a quantitative culture method. In: Research in Burns. H. Huber, Bern, 214.
2. TEN CATE, L. (1965): A note on a simple and rapid method of bacteriological sampling by means of agar sausages. J. appl. Bact. 28 : 221.
3. WAISBREN, B. A., KURZYNSKI, T. A., and MELLENDER, J. W. (1971): Studies of Pseudomonas aeruginosa — the burn pathogen. In: Research in Burns. H. Huber, Bern, 221.

L. P., Legerova 63,
120 00 Praha 2, Czechoslovakia

MAXIMUM TOLERATED DOSES OF GENTAMICIN AND THE SULFAMETHOXAZOLTRIMETHOPRIM-GENTAMICIN COMBINATION IN THE THERAPY OF SEVERE INFECTIONS IN BURNED PATIENTS (PRELIMINARY REPORT)

V. VACEK, R. KÖNIGOVÁ, M. HEJZLAR, T. PELLAR and J. SKŘIVÁNEK

Department of Infectious Diseases, Charles University, Prague, Burns Center, University Hospital, Prague, Military Institute of Microbiology, Prague, Institute of Microbiology, Faculty of Hygiene, Prague, and Medical Faculty, Charles University, Prague, Czechoslovakia

The therapeutic activity of gentamicin in daily doses of 3–5 mg/kg body weight is usually not efficient in septicemias which complicate extensive burns, even when the microbe is sensitive to this antibiotic in the disc test. To improve the therapeutic results in gram-negative infections we investigated the possibility of raising the doses of gentamicin above the recommended limits, up to doses of 10 mg/kg daily. Further, we examined the effectiveness of gentamicin combined with Septrin[R], and the combination of gentamicin with some other antibiotics.

Patients and Methods

All patients were treated at the Burns Center in Prague, and their general condition invariably required intensive care. 46 patients from 3 to 73 years of age were given 58 courses of therapy. In some of them gentamicin was applied twice or three times during the treatment for unrelated infections. The burn of deep second, third and fourth degree involved 20–95 per cent of the body surface. Indication for antibiotics was, most frequently, wound sepsis, bronchopneumonia, and septicemia originating from thrombophlebitis. The bacteriological examination of the burned surface was carried out with the semiquantitative imprint method, and the therapy was designed against the microbes that featured massive growth, i.e. more than 300 colonies on the plate. The sensitivity was determined by disc test. Our study covers only those patients, who received gentamicin in daily doses higher than 5 mg/kg, for at least 3 days, which corresponds to 160–240 mg every 8 hours in adults of average body weight. We analysed 3 groups: the first group was treated with gentamicin only, the second group was treated with the combination of gentamicin and Septrin and the third group received gentamicin plus penicillin derivates or plus lincomycin.

Number of patients, duration of therapy and dosage of gentamicin in single groups are given in Table 1.

In some patients we determined the serum level of gentamicin during the therapy using the standard plate-dilution method. The criterion of a successful therapy was the drop of fever under 38,5 degrees centigrade, subsidence of the overall alteration typical for

TABLE 1

Number of patients duration of therapy and dosage of gentamicin in single groups

Group of patients treated with		gentamicin only	gentamicin + Septrin	gentamicin + other antibiotics
Number of patients Number of gentamicin courses of therapy		18/28–(22/32)*	16/20	12/16
Dose of gentamicin in mg/kg	limits:	5.5–9.0	5.6–9.6	6.0–10.0
	average dose:	7.0	7.3	7.7
Duration of therapy in number of days				
limits:		3.0–15.0	6.0–19.0	3.0–15.0
average:		9.0	9.7	8.0

*) In ten patients who did not respond to gentamicin alone Septrin was added after 2–3 days of gentamicin therapy. Evaluated in the GM/Sm group.

TABLE 2

Results of treatment with gentamicin

Total number of patients	28
Successful therapy	16
Failure	12 (1 died, in 10 patients Septrin added, see next table)
Pathological findings:	bilateral bronchopneumonia nephrosclerosis steatosis of liver

septicemia, disappearing of various organ disturbances, and better condition of burn wound (often suitable for grafting).

Results of treatment

Results of treatment are shown in three separate tables:

Table 2 shows the results of treatment with gentamicin only.

Table 3 shows the results of treatment of 16 patients where gentamicin and Septrin in combination were used.

Table 4 shows the results of treatment with the combination of gentamicin and other antibiotics.

Table 5 shows the serum levels of gentamicin after doses of 240 mg i.m. every 8 hours. We cannot explain the distinctly high levels in the first patient.

Table 6 shows the levels of gentamicin after doses of 240 mg i.m. every eight hours, when given together with oxacillin. The most pressing problem in the treatment with high doses of antibiotics is the frequency, character and gravity of the side-effects.

Table 7 shows the side-effects which appeared in our group of patients during the therapy.

TABLE 3

Results of therapy with combination of gentamicin and Septrin

Total number of patients		16
Successful therapy		9
Failure		7 (all died)
Pathological findings:	1. diabetic glomerulosclerosis bilateral bronchopneumonia Klebsiella bacteriemia	
	2. bilateral bronchopneumonia acute duodenal ulcers pseudomonas + Achromobacter bacteriemia	
	3. bilateral bronchopneumonia lung oedema	
	4. Pseudomonas septicemia (resistent to gentamicin) multiple abscesses in various organs	
	5. bilateral bronchopneumonia focal necroses in myodardium	
	6. bilateral bronchopneumonia lung oedema	
	7. acute tubular necrosis uremia bronchopneumonia lung oedema	

In ten patients where Septrin was added to the unsuccessful gentamicin therapy there were 5 failures and 5 successful cases.

TABLE 4

Results of therapy with combination of gentamicin and other antibiotics

Total number of patients		16
Successful therapy		10
Failure		6 (all died)
Pathological findings:	1. bilateral bronchopneumonia Pseudomonas + E. coli bacteriemia	
	2. bilateral bronchopneumonia subacute glomerulonephritis	
	3. bilateral bronchopneumonia multiple abscesses in kidney and myocardium mucosal lesions in stomach	
	4. bilateral bronchopneumonia Achromobacter bacteriemia subcutaneous abscesses	
	5. bilateral bronchopneumonia Achromobacter bacteriemia bacterial (endotoxin) shock	
	6. lung atelectasis fibrosis of myocardium st. p. endocarditidem	

TABLE 5

Serum levels of gentamicin: single dose 240 mg i.m. applied 8 hourly

Patient	Hours after application of gentamicin				
	1	2	4	6	8
I.R., 65 kg BUN 11.0, Cr 0.9	10.0	16.5	42.0	42.0	33.0
V.Z., 85 kg BUN 16.0, Cr 0.8	14.0	12.8	7.6		4.8
R.N., 80 kg BUN 10.0, Cr 0.3		9.6	6.4	3.2	3.2

Serum levels are given in micrograms/ml

TABLE 6

Serum levels of gentamicin in combination with oxacillin: single dose of gentamicin 240 mg i.m. applied 8 hourly

Patient	Hours after application of gentamicin				
	1	2	4	6	8
J.K., 75 kg BUN 7.0, Cr 0.85 Oxacillin 1 g/4 hrs	1.8	2.7		1.4	
B.P., 80 kg BUN 11.0, Cr 0.6 Oxacillin 2 g/4 hrs	11.0	5.5	1.8		1.4

Serum levels are given in micrograms/ml

TABLE 7

Side-effects of gentamicin (GMC)

Group	GMC only	GMC + Septrin	GMC + other antibiotics	Total
Number of courses of therapy	22	20	16	58
No side effects	13	9	4	26
Renal disturbance already before therapy; no further deterioration after GMC	2	5	3	10
Morbilliform rash	1	0	0	1
Minor changes: proteinuria, haematuria	3	1	4	8
More serious changes (where BUN or Cr were elevated)	3	3	5	11
Positive liver function tests	0	1	0	1
Partial loss of hearing, BUN + serum creatinine increased	0	1	0	1

Discussion

After two and a half years of treatment with higher doses of gentamicin up to 720 mg daily, we feel that it has conclusively helped to improve the therapeutic results. The overall tolerance of injections was good.

As regards the gentamicin-Septrin group, although half of the treated patients died, this combination can hardly be described as antagonistic. This group includes 10 patients, in whom the therapy with gentamicin alone failed to produce any improvement after 2–4 days, and who received Septrin, because potentiation was expected. Five of them died and five were successful. The effectivity of this combination was very marked in burns of respiratory tract connected with tracheostomy, in bronchopneumonias, and in mixed infection of burn wound, where Staphylococcus aureus, sensitive to Septrin, was present. Gentamicin alone, even in high doses, evidently cannot eradicate massive Staphylococcus infections, even with proved sensitivity.

In the third group, gentamicin was applied together with other antibiotics. In one case the combination with penicillin G in a dose of 20 millions units daily was successful even in Achromobacter septicemia, the strain being resistent to gentamicin in disc test. Combination with oxacillin was used mostly in mixed infections, where Staphylococcus aureus or beta-hemolytic streptococci prevailed. Combination with lincomycin was effective in multiple subcutaneous abscesses, where heterografting was protected. The choice of the antibiotic against Staphylococci depends on the sentitivity, but the antibiotics mentioned above, have been used most frequently.

Side-Effects

More than one third of the patients suffered from side-effects, mostly reversible changes in urine and in serum demonstrating certain degree of nephrotoxicity (erythrocyturia, proteinuria, increase of BUN and serum creatinine).

The findings were of minor clinical importance, except in two cases. In survivors, the pathological findings subsided within two weeks after discontinuation of treatment. The incidence was most marked in patients who received gentamicin together with penicillin derivatives, whereas no significant differences were found between the gentamicin and gentamicin-septrin groups. One case with impaired liver function was most probably related to the organ disturbances during burn illness. The partial loss of hearing in one case was caused by overdosage, when lowering the doses lagged behind the development of renal impairment. In another case we started gentamicin immediately after the shock period, and gentamicin very probably worsened the renal damage. We must be careful in indicating higher doses of gentamicin in the cases, in which the kidney has not yet completely recovered from shock. On the contrary, even high doses of gentamicin caused no further deterioration of renal function in those patients, in whom the pathological findings in urine of other than shock origin existed already before starting treatment. These ten cases were recorded separately, as it was difficult to ascertain if gentamicin caused further changes of minor character or not. Setting the risk of the observed toxic side-effects against high danger of gram-negative septicemia in extensive burns, we consider the therapy with high doses of gantamicin justified in all respects, but intensive care of the patient is a must. We recommend daily urine, BUN, serum creatinine, and hearing ability checks.

As far as necropsy findings are concerned, in the majority of patients who died, the bronchopneumonia was the main cause of death. There were several cases of uncontrolable septicemia as well, and some of the causative agents were resistant to gentamicin. Only in one case the microscopical examination of kidneys revealed changes that might be attributable to gentamicin toxicity.

Blood levels of gentamicin

Because only few results are available at present no analysis is possible. We are going to discuss this subject in a separate paper.

CONCLUSION

We present the first experiences with gentamicin in daily doses of 5–10 mg/kg, administered alone, or in combination with other antibiotics in the therapy of septicemia in severe burns. Our therapeutic results are encouraging, and appear to justify this tactic, despite somewhat higher incidence of undesirable side-effects.

V. V., Dept. of Infectious Dis.,
Bulovka Hospital,
180 81 Praha 8, Czechoslovakia

FREQUENCY OF SEPTICAEMIA

M. THOMSEN

Burns Unit, Copenhagen, Denmark

As early as 1933 Aldrich (1) at the Johns Hopkins hospital in USA demonstrated streptococci in the wounds and cardiac blood of fatally burned patients, and two years later Cruickshank (4) in Scotland isolated haemolytic streptococci from the spleen and endocardium of patients who had died of burns.

Ten years later Colebrook et al. (3) in Glasgow had only one death from septicaemia due to haemolytic streptococci in their series from the Burns Unit 1942–43, but in 1954 Liedberg, Reiss and Artz (5) from the Brooke Army Medical Center in Texas showed that in their series septicaemia was a common cause of death in burns. In Liedberg's opinion many unexplained deaths after burns were due to septicaemia, and many cases excaped diagnosis because the patients survived.

During the 1950ies the predominant microorganism changed from staphylococci to Pseudomonas and the mortality figures rose considerably. The clinical picture of the gram-negative septicaemia was intensively studied by burn surgeons and Moncrief and Teplitz (7) discussed the difficulties of isolating the Pseudomonas bacteria. Stone et al. (8), described verdoglobinuria as a sign of Pseudomonas septicaemia and its prognostic role, and Lindberg et al. (6) from the Brooke Army Medical Center demonstrated an increasing incidence of septicaemia as a consequence of an increasing number of extensive burns, and an amazingly high mortality.

The pathologist Teplitz et al. (9) have demonstrated that as early as four days after inoculation with Pseudomonas into experimental burns, healthy tissue in the depth will be invaded, whereas staphylococci, though spreading in the wounds, do not invade vital tissue. Pseudomonas is disseminated especially along the vessels and may be demonstrated in perivascular infiltrations.

In the Burns Unit in Copenhagen we have studied the frequency of clinical infection in burns and its dependence upon the size of the burns and the age of the patients (10). In Fig. 1 the findings have been illustrated in a diagrammatic form. The patients have been divided into four groups of age from top to bottom, and into five groups by area of burn from left to right. The dark sectors of the circles indicate the percentage of patients with clinical infection in the group concerned. It is clearly demonstrated that the frequency of the infection increases with increasing age of the patients and with increasing area of their burns. In elderly patients and in major burns the frequency of clinical infection is thus 100 per cent, and this dependence upon the age of the patients and the extent of their burns is strikingly reminiscent of the mortality figures shown by Bull and Squire (2) as early as 25 years ago.

In Fig. 2 the rate of clinical infection in the same patients is shown for various areas of burns, divided into deep and superficial lesions. It is apparent that there is a distinct

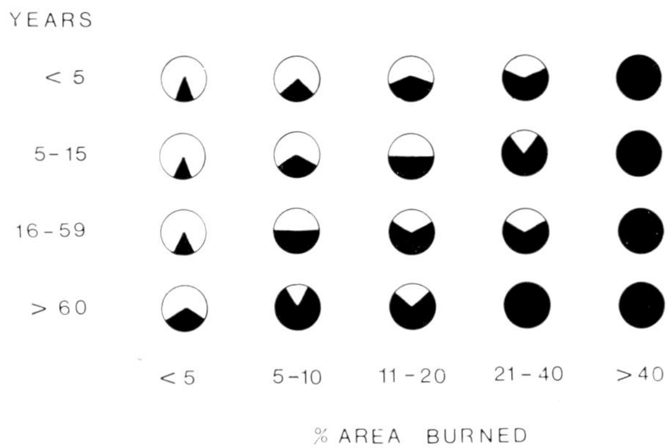

Fig. 1. Percentage of patients with clinical infection in dependence on age and size of burned area (black segments)

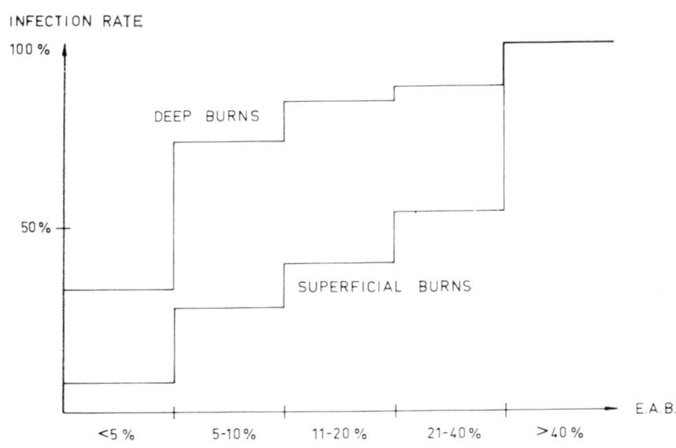

Fig. 2. Infection rate in dependence on the size of burned area and depth of burns.

difference between the two curves except in very extensive burns where all get infected regardless of the depth of their burns.

We thus find an increasing rate of infection in burns with increasing area and depth of the burns as well as by increasing ages of the patients. And now to the bacteriology.

Fig. 3 shows you the frequency of infection with Pseudomonas at various ages of the patients with clinical infection. The patients have been divided into the same groups of ages as previously, i.e. infants, school-children, adults, and elderly patients more than 60 years of age. It is apparent that the frequency of infection with Pseudomonas increases with increasing ages of the patients.

Even more striking is this dependence, when we consider the frequency of infection with Pseudomonas at various areas of burns. In Fig. 4 the burns have been divided into the same five groups of areas as previously, and it is clearly demonstrated that the infection with Pseudomonas is increasing with increasing areas of the burns. As a matter of fact this microorganism occurs forty times as often in burns exceeding 40 per cent of body surface than in small burns, less than 5 per cent of body surface.

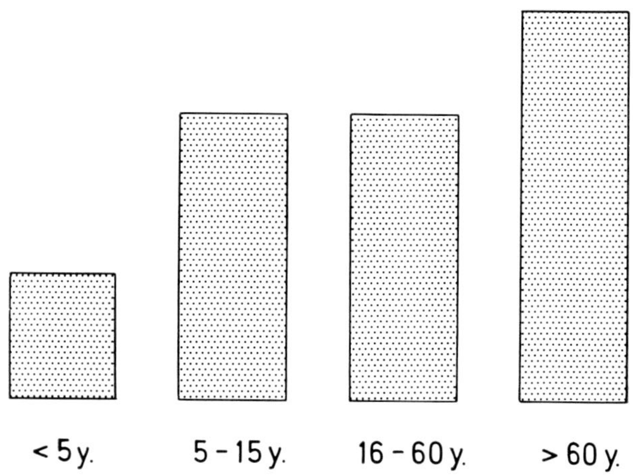

Fig. 3. Frequency of Ps. aeruginosa at various ages.

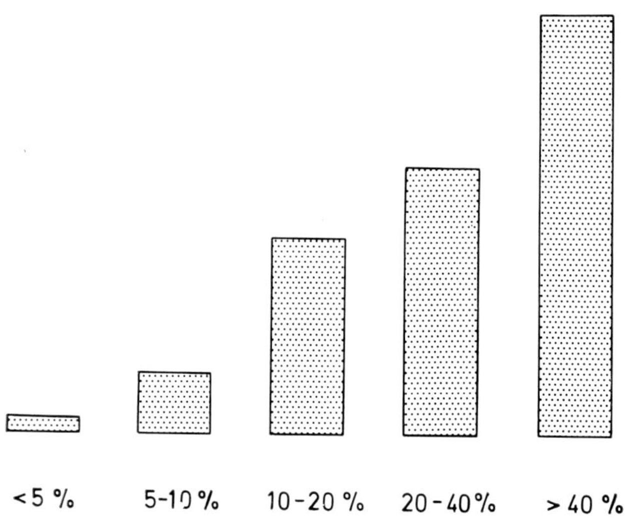

Fig. 4. Ps. aeruginosa at various areas of burns.

Fig. 5 shows you the difference of the frequency of infection with Pseudomonas in superficial and deep burns, regardless of the area and the age of the patients. Again you see an enormous difference between the two groups, and these facts also concern most of the other bacteria which belong to the group of the gram-negatives (11).

And now finally to septicaemia.

In the Burns Unit in Copenhagen this syndrom occurred almost exclusively in cases with deep burns exceeding 20 per cent of body surface, and in patients over 60 years of

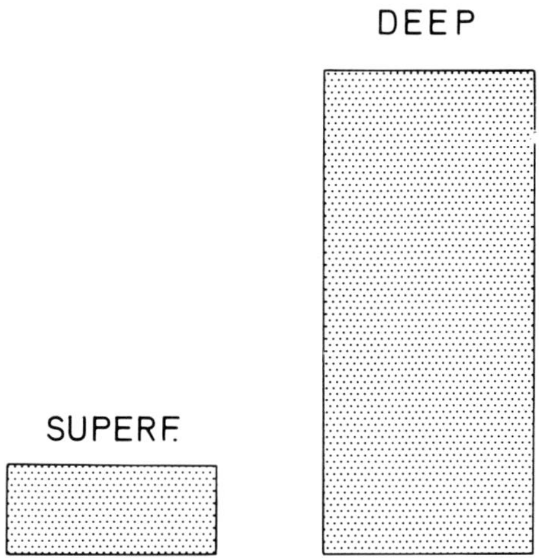

Fig. 5. Frequency of Ps. aeruginosa in deep and superficial burns.

age (12). The mortality was very high in cases of septicaemia with gram-negative bacteria, whereas all patients with staphylococci in the blood survived. In most instances the bacteria isolated from the blood were also present in the burn wounds.

In conclusion we can say that it is old patients and patients with very extensive and deep burns who run the greatest risk of getting a septicaemia. It is also this category of patients who has the greatest frequency of clinical infection, and their burns are predominated by a gram-negative bacterial flora. These factors have only seldom been taken into consideration in discussing the frequency of septicaemia in burns, but nevertheless they might give us one of the keys to a solution of the problem.

References

1. Aldrich, R. H. (1933): The role of infection in burns. New Engl. J. Med. 208 : 299.
2. Bull, J. P. and Squire, J. R. (1949): A study of mortality in a Burns Unit. Ann. Surg. 130 : 160.
3. Colebrook, L., Clark, A. M., Gibson, T. and Todd, J. P. (1945): The control of infection in burns and scalds. In: Studies of burns and scalds (ed. Med. Res. Counc.), part II, p. 17. His Maj. Stat. Office, London.
4. Cruickshank, R. (1935): The bacterial infection of burns. J. Path. Bact. 41 : 367.
5. Liedberg, C. F., Reis, E. and Artz, C. P. (1954): Infection in burns. III. Septicaemia, a common cause of death. Surg. Gynec. Obstet. 99 : 151.
6. Lindberg, R. B., Moncrief, J. A. and Mason, A. D. (1968): Control of experimental and clinical burn wound sepsis by topical application of Sulfamylon compounds. Ann. N.Y. Acad. Sci. 150 : 950.

7. MONCRIEF, J. A. and TEPLITZ, C. (1964): Changing concepts in burn sepsis. J. Trauma 4 : 233.
8. STONE, H. H., MARTIN, J. D. and GRABER, C. D. (1964): Verdoglobinuria: an ominous sign of pseudomonas septicemia in burns. Ann. Surg. 159 : 994.
9. TEPLITZ, C., DAVIS, D., MASON, A. D. JR. and MONCRIEF, J. A. (1964): Pseudomonas burn wound sepsis. I. Pathogenesis of experimental burn wound sepsis. J. surg. Res. 4 : 200.
10. THOMSEN, M. (1970): The Burns Unit in Copenhagen. VI. Infection rates. Scand. J. plast. reconstr. Surg. 4 : 53.
11. THOMSEN, M. (1970): The Burns Unit in Copenhagen. VIII. Bacteriology. Scand. J. plast. reconstr. Surg. 4 : 126.
12. THOMSEN, M. (1970): The Burns Unit in Copenhagen. IX. Occurrence of septicaemia 1961—1968. Scand. J. plast. reconstr. Surg. 4 : 141.

M. T., Bueager 7,
2950 Vedbaek, Denmark

PHAGOCYTIC PROPERTIES OF LEUKOCYTES IN BURNS

J. W. ALEXANDER, A. McCLELLAN, E. S. LENNARD
and A. BUNDEALLY

Department of Surgery, University of Cincinnati Medical Center and the Shriners Burns Institute, Cincinnati, Ohio 45229, U.S.A.

Infection continues to be the leading cause of death following burn injury. Since neutrophils are an essential component of resistance to bacterial infections, a variety of tests have been performed to evaluate their function in patients with major thermal injury.

Materials and Methods

Patient Population

Two series of patients with major burn injuries were studied. The first series (A), studied between 1968 and 1971, consisted of 48 patients with an average age of 15.6 years and an average total burn of 53.6 per cent (1). The second series of 14 patients (B) was studied during the last year and had an average age of 20.3 years and an average burn size of 58.7 per cent.

Test of Neutrophil Function

A standardized test was used for the measurement of the antibacterial function of neutrophils using *S. aureus 502A* (1). A total of 573 tests were performed in series A patients and 135 tests in series B patients over a total of 1972 days of patient observation. Therefore, each patient was studied an average of 11.4 times during 32 days. Sixty-seven tests of neutrophil function using *E. coli* as the test organism were done concurrently in the last 6 patients. Also run concurrently in series B patients were serial tests to measure migration of neutrophils and the chemotactic response of neutrophils to endotoxin.

Results

The antibacterial function of neutrophils was expressed as a neutrophil-bactericidal index (NBI) which compared the function of a patient's neutrophils with the average function of neutrophils from 2–5 normal controls (1). The average NBI for burn patients in series A was 5.7, indicating a rather severe deficiency. In contrast, the average NBI for

Supported by USPHS Grant ≠ 5PO-1-GM15428-06.

series B patients was 1.64, indicative of only a mild dysfunction. The average NBI for *E. coli* in the last six patients in series B was −0.44, indicating a completely normal neutrophil function for this organism. In series A, the average neutrophil bactericidal index associated with the onset of sepsis was 15.9 compared to only 2.03 in series B (P less than 0.01). This dramatic difference in average neutrophil function between series A and B has been associated with a significant fall in the rate of sepsis and an increase in the burn survival as measured by the LA_{50} (Table 1). Of all patients with burn injuries greater than 20 per cent admitted during the time series A patients were being studied, 39.3 per cent had positive blood cultures at some time during their hospital course. Of all patients with greater than 20 per cent burn admitted during the time that series B patients were studied, only 33.7 per cent had positive blood cultures. Random migration of leukocytes in series B patients was often depressed, but had no direct correlation with either septic episodes or the antibacterial function of neutrophils. Likewise, the chemotactic response to endotoxin in Boyden chambers was significantly depressed in series B patients, but the degree of depression was not correlated with septic episodes nor was it correlated significantly with the antibacterial function of neutrophils.

TABLE 1

Series	Number of Patients	Average NBI	Total Episodes of Sepsis	Average NBI of Onset of Sepsis	Incidence of Bacteremia in all Patients with Burns > 20 per cent Admitted Same Approximate Period	LA_{50}
A	48	5.7	45	15.9	39.3 % of 239 Patients	65
B	14	1.46	8	2.03	33.7 % of 83 Patients	72

In series A patients, depression of neutrophil function was clearly associated with septic episodes, and patients who had septic episodes had significantly higher NBI values than those who did not (P less than 0.005). Also, the average NBI at the onset of sepsis was significantly higher than the average for the tests obtained from the same patients when they were not septic (P less than 0.005). In these patients, the abnormalities of neutrophilic function clearly preceeded the onset of septic episodes. Cyclic variation of neutrophil function was observed in both series of patients. Septic episodes in series B patients occurred on 8 occasions, but only two episodes were related to poor neutrophil function; four were related to defects in serum opsonins, and two could not be explained.

Abnormal neutrophil function in burn patients was associated with an increase in the rate of phagocytosis and a diminution in the intracellular killing of bacteria. At no time was there evidence of an intrinsic defect in phagocytosis in burn neutrophils. Studies using lysostaphin to disrupt staphylococci in the extracellular medium of the tests indicated that all of the viable bacteria were intracellular after a 4 hour incubation period, further indicating that the defect in antibacterial killing was intracellular rather than an inability to phagocytize bacteria. Bacterial multiplication within phagocytic vacoules was clearly evidenced by electron microscopy. Sequential studies showed that killing by burn neutrophils in series A patients was essentially normal during the first 30 minutes, but killing was arrested after 60 minutes. In both series A and B patients, there was clear evidence that cyclic variations in the antibacterial function for different strains of bacteria was not necessarily correlated, indicating that there are different mechanisms of intracellular killing for these different organisms.

Discussion

The tests of neutrophilic antibacterial function described herein measure a significant component of host resistance which has been found to be abnormal in many patients with serious burn injury. These acquired abnormalities contribute significantly to the onset of infection in burned patients, and the degree of abnormality has been significantly associated with the incidence and seriousness of septic episodes.

A striking difference in the average antibacterial function of neutrophils has been found between patients in series A and series B, with much better function being present in the latter group. Associated with this improvement in neutrophil function has been a reduction in the rate and seriousness of infection. However, the factors responsible for this improvement are not entirely clear since basic management has not changed except for a more aggressive approach to early removal of the burn eschar and an improvement of the nutritional status via dietary supplementation. It is uncertain at the present time which of these has contributed more to the improvement in neutrophilic antibacterial function, but other evidence would suggest that nutritional factors were largely responsible. As an example, kwashiorkor and iron deficiency anemia are both associated with abnormalities of neutrophil function. However, in our laboratory, we have been unable to produce defects of neutrophil function by acute starvation.

Summary

The antibacterial function of neutrophils in patients with severe thermal injury may be significantly depressed. When abnormal function occurs, it is often associated with the onset of sepsis, and increasing degrees of abnormality are associated with an increasing incidence of septic episodes. The abnormality appears to be associated with a nutritional defect since more recent patients with a better nutritional status and dietary supplementation had improved neutrophilic function.

References

1. Alexander, J. W. and Meakins, J. L. (1972): A physiological basis for the development of opportunistic infections in man. Ann. Surg. 176 : 273.

J. W. A., Dept. of Surgery,
Cincinnati General Hosp.,
Cincinnati, Ohio 45229, U.S.A.

IMMUNOTHERAPY IN BURNS

J. W. ALEXANDER

Department of Surgery, University of Cincinnati Medical Center, Cincinnati, Ohio 45229, and the Cincinnati Shriners Burns Institute, U.S.A.

Major thermal injury is associated with a significant susceptibility to life-threatening infections. Prominent among these have been infections caused by *Pseudomonas aeruginosa*, a ubiquitous pathogen which rarely causes disease in healthy individuals. However, in patients with thermal injury, host defenses are compromised by a number of mechanisms, susceptibility to Pseudomonas is increased, and infections caused by this microorganism often progress rapidly. Despite many recent advances in therapy, septic death continues to occur from Pseudomonas at the rate of 5 to 15 per cent in patients with burns involving greater than 20 per cent total body surface area.

In an effort to control this pathogen, a series of immunological studies were begun in 1964, which have resulted in clinical and laboratory investigations of a heptavalent Pseudomonas vaccine (2), (Pseudogen[R], Parke-Davis and Co.) and a hyperimmune anti-Pseudomonas globulin (4) for immunotherapy against *Pseudomonas* in burn injury. This vaccine has now been used continuously at the University of Cincinnati for five years, and this report summarizes the clinical results of this experience.

MATERIALS AND METHODS

This study included 332 vaccinated patients with burn injuries involving greater than 20 per cent of the total body surface area admitted between March, 1968, and April, 1973. Since these were the initial studies of this vaccine in humans, a variety of routes and doses for administration of the immunogen were evaluated. However, the patients could be divided into three basic groups. The first 40 patients received a low dose vaccination that was considered to be suboptimal. The next 96 patients received optimal vaccination consisting of 25 micron/kg/injection for up to 10 injections. The final 186 patients also received optimal vaccination and, in addition, a hyperimmune anti-Pseudomonas gammaglobulin was utilized for the treatment of patients who developed active Pseudomonas sepsis. Comparison of the effectiveness of immunotherapy was made among these three

---

Supported by a grant from Parke-Davis and Company, Detroit, Michigan and U.S. Army Contract ≠ DA-49-193-MD2531.

TABLE 1

Comparison of patient data

Phases of Study	Number of Patients	Dates Mo/yr	Average Age	Av. Size Burn Total/ 3rd degree	Burn Index	Positive Blood Cultures Other than Ps. (per cent)	Deaths All Causes (per cent)	LA_{50} (per cent)
Control	75	1/67/3/68	12.3	39.2/27.7	33.5	42.7	26.7	55
I & II Suboptimal dose and route	40	3/68–2/69	14.1	42.8/26.9	34.8	42.5	20.0	60
III Optimal dose, no globulin	96	2/69–7/70	14.6	42.8/28.3	35.5	39.2	21.7	63
IV–VI Optimal dose plus globulin for sepsis	186	7/70/4/73	19.5	42.5/25.9	34.2	36.0	22.6	72

TABLE 2

Efect of Immunotherapy on Pseudomonas Infection. Patients who developed Pseudomonas septicemia within five days after starting immunization or who died from any cause during the first five days of hospitalization were exluded

Phases of Study	Number of Patients	Colonization by Ps. aeruginosa (per cent)	Positive Blood Cultures Pseudomonas (per cent)	Deaths from Pseudomonas (per cent)
Control	75	72.2	18.7	14.7
I and II	40	72.5	15.0	12.5
III	96	73.2	8.3	3.1
IV–VI	186	66.1	5.9	0.0

groups and with a group of 75 consecutive similarly burned non-vaccinated patients treated at our institution between January, 1967, and March, 1968. A comparison of patient data is shown in Table 1.

Results

The results of the immunotherapy program against *Pseudomonas aeruginosa* are shown in Table 2. Immunization did not significantly decrease the rate of colonization of patients with *Pseudomonas aeruginosa* as evidenced by recovery of a positive culture from any site. In contrast, vaccination selectively decreased the number of positive blood cultures for *Pseudomonas* to a significant degree, and deaths caused by infection from *Pseudomonas aeruginosa* were markedly decreased. It is noteworthy that among the last 186 severely burned patients who did not become septic during the initial 5 days after immunization was begun, no deaths occurred from *Pseudomonas aeruginosa* although *Pseudomonas* septicemia occurred in 10 of these patients. This favorable survival was possible largely from the availability and use of anti-Pseudomonas hyperimmune globulin for the treatment of vaccine failures. The dosage of the globulin and more complete data concerning its use are detailed in a previous report(4).

During the study, approximately 3000 injections of the vaccine were given. Almost 1/2 of the injections caused some detectable local or systemic response as evidenced by induration, tenderness, or a temperature elevation, but none of these reactions were considered to be serious. However, in a few patients, the dosage of the vaccine was decreased or even discontinued because of local or febrile response.

Discussion

This large clinical experience is subject to criticism because it does not represent a randomized double blind study, and the controls were not concurrent with the patients who received immunization. Yet, the results are extremely impressive and leave little doubt for those who have been associated with the study that preventive immunization with the vaccine and active therapy with the hyperimmune globulin can provide significant protection against septic death caused by *Pseudomonas aeruginosa*. The gradual improvement in survival and the more impressive increase in the LA_{50} of burn injury during the successive periods of vaccination appear to result largely from control of lethal *Pseudomonas* infections. Our results in burn patients are similar to the results of effectiveness which have been shown in a controlled prospective study for the protection of cancer patients against *Pseudomonas* infection. (5)

These studies have also led to an appreciation that the IgG type of antibody rather than the IgM provides the major protection against infection from *Pseudomonas aeruginosa* (1). Further analysis has shown that immune IgG antibody is far more effective than natural IgG antibody since it does not require participation of the alternate pathway of complement which is often abnormal after burn injury (3).

Summary

Three hundred twenty-two patients with burn injuries involving 20 per cent or more total body surface area have been actively vaccinated with a polyvalent Pseudomonas vaccine at our center during the five year period preceding April, 1973. Optimal high dose vaccination has resulted in a decrease in Pseudomonas bacteriemia from 18.7 to 5.9 per cent. In those patients who did not develop Pseudomonas sepsis during the first five days after immunization was begun, death from Pseudomonas was decreased by optimal vaccination alone to 3.1 compared to 14.7 per cent in a similar control group. Deaths caused by *Pseudomonas aeruginosa* infection have not occurred in the last 186 patients in whom the vaccination procedure has been supplemented by the administration of anti-Pseudomonas hyperimmune globulin to patients who developed septicemia by clinical and laboratory criteria. These results strongly support the use of this and similar vaccines for the prevention and control of sepsis following burn injury.

References

1. Alexander, J. W. and Fisher, M. W. (1970): Immunological determinants of Pseudomonas infections of man accompanying severe burn injury. J. Trauma 10 : 565.
2. Alexander, J. W., Fisher, M. W. and MacMillan, B. G. (1971): Immunological control of Pseudomonas infection in burn patients: A clinical evaluation. Arch. Surg. 102 : 31.
3. Bjornson, A. B. and Alexander, J. W.: Alterations of serum opsonins in patients with severe thermal injury (Submitted for publication).
4. Jones, C. E., Alexander, J. W. and Fisher, M. W. (1973): Clinical evaluation of Pseudomonas hyperimmune globulin. J. surg. Res. 14 : 87.
5. Young, L. S., Meyers, R. D. and Armstrong, D.: Pseudomonas aeruginosa vaccine in cancer patients. Report of a controlled prospective trial. Ann. inter. Med. (To be published).

J. W. A., Dept. of Surgery,
Cincinnati General Hosp.,
Cincinnati, Ohio 45229, U.S.A.

THE ROLE OF THE RETICULOENDOTHELIAL SYSTEM IN BURN INFECTION

G. LEMPERLE

Clinic for Plastic and Reconstructive Surgery, St. Marcus Hospital, Frankfurt, F.R.G.

Bacteriemia is a daily event in a healthy person and occurs even after chewing and tooth brushing. Its harmlessness is caused by the host defense system which includes specific and nonspecific serum antibodies and the macrophages of the reticuloendothelial system (RES). Ninety percent of these macrophages are located in the liver as so-called Kupffer cells, lining the sinusoids like a three dimensional filter. There are twice as many endothelial cells as hepatocytes in the liver, but they are less obvious since their volume is 20 times less than that of a hepatocyte. Under normal conditions only approximately 40 per cent of the RE-cells are active, i.e. phagocytizing and detoxifying, while the other 60 per cent are resting until a stimulant or irritant such as trauma, tumor-growth, infection or a certain drug increases their activity.

The broad spectrum of reticuloendothelial functions include the phagocytosis of bacteria, cell fragments, fibrin clots and toxic substances, a step in antibody formation, the synthesis and conjugation of certain steroids, the hydrolysis of cholesterol and the neutralization of enzymes as well as an important step in fat and iron metabolism and in the removal of certain blood clotting factors. One has to look upon these different parameters of the RES as a whole, in order to understand the effects of stimulation or depression on other biological functions.

After a severe burn injury, all of these parameters are markedly impaired and can be blocked by the least additional burden. The depression of phagocytic and detoxifying mechanisms appears to be due to the liberation of endotoxin-like materials from the gut and from the burned area (10). Despite early recovery of phagocytic activity after burn shock, men and experimental animals seem to have lost the ability to react adequately to the stimulus of infection. This is due to a depletion of opsonins from the serum (1, 9) as well as to an impaired capacity for intracellular destruction (3, 4). While gram-negative bacteria have to be opsonized by specific antibody gram-positive bacteria are rapidly phagocytized by the RE-cells, obviously without specific opsonization. The intracellular breakdown of gram-negative bacteria, however, does not necessarily include detoxification of the liberated endotoxin molecules (4) which appears to be a problem especially in burn shock. On the other hand, cortisone exerts its benificial effect in the shock period by stabilizing the lysosomal membranes towards these intracellularly liberated toxins (3).

In order to get an insight into these rather complicated events after burn injury and to find the cause of the lack of host defense mechanisms in burn patients, one parameter of the RES, its phagocytic activity, was determined with the aid of the Carbon-Clearance-Test in animals (2) and the Lipofundin-Clearance-Test in human patients (8). A certain amount of carbon particles in the form of India ink or of lipid droplets in the form of a fat emulsion is injected intravenously and its clearance rate from the blood is determined spectrophotometrically. In the past 10 years our main interest concentrated on drugs and other therapeutic regimen in burned patients which may have a depressing or stimulating effect on phagocytosis.

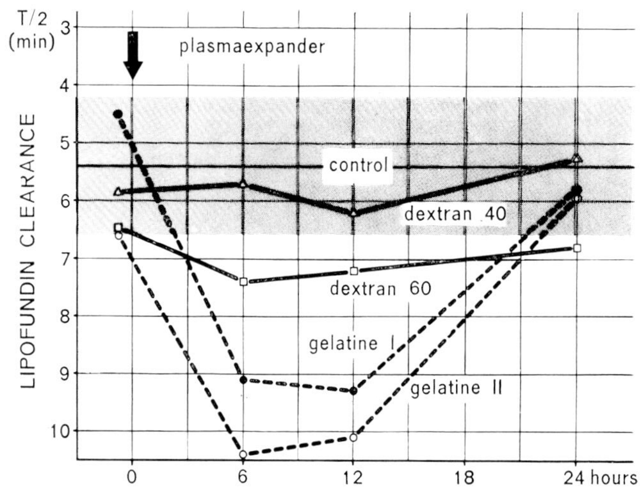

Fig. 1. Lipofundin-Clearance-Test in 62 blood donors after replacement of 500 ml blood by 500 ml plasma substitute.

In animal experiments we could demonstrate that certain antibiotics which were widely used in prophylaxis of postburn infection exerted a depressing effect on phagocytosis (7). At present, however, chloramphenicol and tetracyclines are abandoned in most burn units in favour of more effective antibiotics such as gentamycin, cephalothin or ampicillin. These latter do not interfere with protein synthesis in bacteria and mammalian cells as well; therefore, they do not impair phagocytosis and antibody production in the host.

On the other hand, plasma substitutes on gelatin and dextran base were shown to have a depressing effect on phagocytosis in mice (7). We could confirm these results in healthy human blood donors replacing 500 ml blood with 500 ml dextran or gelatin fluid (Fig. 1). Two gelatin preparations (Haemaccel = gelatin II and Neo-Plasmagel = gelatin I) effected a significant depression of phagocytosis over 18 hours which was not due to physical overloading of the RES but probably due to a depletion or precipitation of opsonins.

Another group of substances is in daily use on a burn ward: anesthetics and analgesics. Postoperative RE-depression has been found to be closely related to the narcotic substance and the duration of narcosis whereas the operative stress alone caused little alteration of phagocytic activity. Fluothane and barbiturates exerted a marked RE-depression in mice, which underwent a one-hour-narcosis. Pentrane, ether and nitrous oxide, on the other hand, did not effect RE function (Fig. 2). These findings could be confirmed in human patients (8) who also demonstrated their strongest inhibition in the first 6 hours after narcosis.

A single injection of morphine depressed phagocytosis in mice for 6 hours, while the injection of a morphine derivative was followed by an increased activity. Some of the newer strong analgesics: Fortral, Dipidolor and Valoron coused phagocytic depression while tranquillizers such as Valium f.i. exerted no effect on the RES. As with all biologically effective drugs, small doses often caused a stimulation, high doses a depression

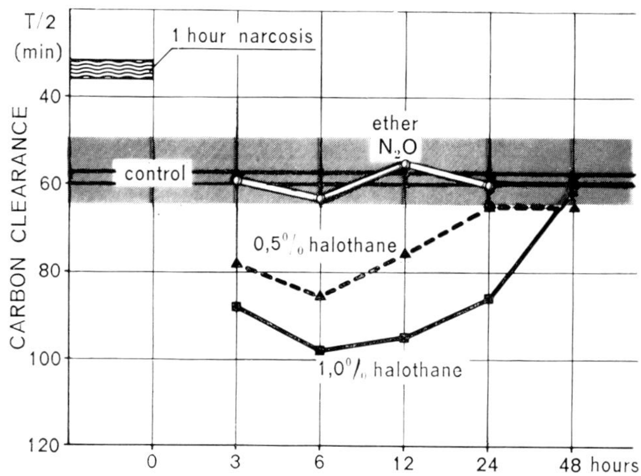

Fig. 2. One hour narcosis with fluothane caused RE-depression which lasted up to 24 hours in mice.

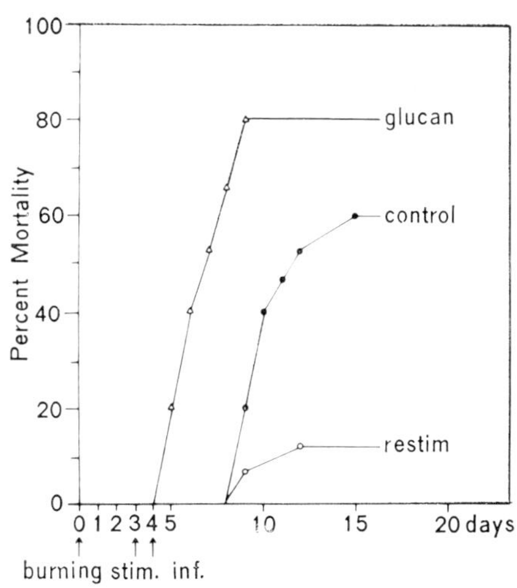

Fig. 3. Postburn mortality in rats after RE-stimulation with restim or glucan on day 3 and infection with Ps. aeruginosa on day 4.

or vice versa, i.e. all results of clearance tests have to be looked upon as being strictly dose dependent.

In view of a prospective therapy of postburn RE-depression and therewith prevention of septicaemia RES — stimulants have to be mentioned which have been found very effective in experimental cancer, shock and postburn infections (6, 7). So far, they were mainly of theoretical interest for human patients, since most of them effect granuloma formation in the liver, spleen and lungs, and only BCG — vaccination has been considered for a clinical trial in leucaemic patients. Another potent stimulant in animal experiments, however, the shark liver lipid Restim was especially effective in gram-negative infection (67) and endotoxin shock (Fig. 3), while Glucan, an extract from yeast cell wall rendered RE cells rather susceptible to Ps. aeruginosa endotoxin.

What might look like a promising therapy in the postburn period is opsonin, which recently has been isolated with a 100-fold purification (1). It is an alpha-globulin and can be stored in a lyophilized state with retention of all biological activity. This can lead to an intravenous opsonin therapy in patients with an opsonin — mediated RE depression e.g. during tumor surgery and after severe trauma or burn injury.

Conclusion

Phagocytic activity and opsonin production are greatly impaired after shock and severe burn injury. Inadequate postburn therapy with certain antibiotics, plasma substitutes and analgesics may further depress the exhausted functions of the RES. Thus, septicaemia occurs and overwhelms host defense mechanisms. A well-functioning RES appears to be the prerequisite for an effective antibiotic therapy and should therefore be considered in all prescriptions to burn patients. The use of RES-stimulants in combination with opsonin therapy will hopefully become an effective treatment for postburn infection.

References

1. Allen, Ch., Saba, T. M. and Molnar, J. (1973): Isolation, purification and characterization of opsonic protein. J. Reticuloendothel. Soc. 13 : 410.
2. Benacerraf, B., Thorbecke, G. J., Jacoby, D. (1959): Effect of zymosan on endotoxin toxicity in mice. Proc. Soc. exper. Biol. (N.Y.) 100 : 796.
3. Bengmark, S., Fredlund, P. E., Kallum, B. et al. (1973): The effect of corticosteroids on the release of lysosomal enzymes in liver ischaemia and shock. Europ. Surg. Res. 5, Suppl. 1 : 73.
4. Filkins, J. P. (1973): Acidic pH and the hepatic detoxification of endotoxin. J. Reticuloendothel. Soc. 11 : 293.
5. Lemperle, G. (1966): Effect of RES stimulation on endotoxin shock in mice. Proc. Soc. exp. Biol. (N.Y.). 122 : 1012.
6. Lemperle, G. (1967): Stimulation of the reticuloendothelial sytem in burned rats infected with Ps. aeruginosa. J. infect. Dis. 117 : 7.
7. Lemperle, G. (1970): Depression and stimulation of host defense mechanisms after severe burn injury. Plast. reconstr. Surg. 45 : 435.
8. Lemperle, G. and Reichelt, M. (1973): Der Lipofundin-Clearance-Test, ein Maß für die Phagocytose-Aktivität des RES. Med. Klinik 68 : 48.
9. Schildt, B. E. and Bouveng, R. (1971): Effect of burning on hepatic phagocytosis as studied in vitro. Life Sci. 10 : 397.
10. Städtler, K., Allgöwer, M., Cueni, L. B. and Schönenberger, G. A. (1972): Formation of a specific "burn toxin" in mouse skin by thermal injury. Europ. Surg. Res. 4 : 198.

G. L., St. Markus-Hosp.,
6000 Frankfurt 50, F.R.G.

A STUDY ON THE APPEARANCE OF AUTO-IMMUNE PHENOMENA IN BURN PATIENTS AND ITS CLINICAL RELEVANCE

P. LEGUIT, JR.

University Clinic of Surgery, Binnengasthuis, Amsterdam, The Netherlands

INTRODUCTION

Thermal trauma is thought to cause changes in the structure of body components. The slightly altered auto-antigens might no longer be recognized as "self" by the immune system thus leading to the production of autoantibodies which may cross-react with the original native structure. As full thickness burn injuries consist of a trauma of all layers of the epidermis and sometimes involve skeletal muscle, bones, joints and even lungs, the appearance of auto-immune reaction to all these tissue components seems feasible.

After thermal injury antibodies have been observed both in experimental animals and in man against the antigens of red blood cells (6), white blood cells (10, 18), nuclei (10, 19), basement membrane of skin (20), collagen (5), immunoglobulins (10, 11, 19) and skin (8, 9, 17, 19, 20, 21).

A study of auto-antibodies is of particular importance, since some pathological conditions have been attributed to these antibodies. For instance it has been claimed by Eastern literature that anaemia following burn trauma might partly be due to the appearance of erythrocyte antibodies (6). Renal function is seen to be influenced, which might be due to the appearance of kidney-antibodies (13).

RESULTS

In the present study 79 sera from 23 patients with burns ranging from 10 do 90 per cent of the total body surface were studied at two weeks intervals post burn.

Table 1 gives a survey of the auto-antibodies studied, the methods used, and the mere results. Our investigations were negative for most antigens:

1. Using the direct anti-globulin test with different anti-globulin sera we did not find any positive reactions when studying erythrocyte antibodies.

These studies were performed in the Central Laboratory of the Netherland Red Cross Blood Transfusion Service and the Laboratory of Experimental and Clinical Immunology of the University of Amsterdam, Holland.

TABLE 1

Appearance of (auto)-antibodies in burned patients (n = 23)

Antigen	Method	Result
erythrocyte	direct antiglobulin test	—
leucocyte	cytotoxicity, agglutination	—
kidney	passive haemagglutination	—
nuclei	immunofluorescence technique (=IFT)	—
stomach	IFT	—
smooth muscle	IFT	—
skeletal muscle	IFT	—
mitochondria	IFT	—
salivary gland	IFT	—
thyroid	IFT	—
immunoglobulin	passive haemagglutination, haemagglutination-inhibition	+ (n=3)
skin	IFT	+ (n=8)

2. In contrast to recent Western reports (10, 18, 19) we did not find antileukocyte antibodies and anti-nuclear antibodies.

3. It was thought that in the view of the known existence of common antigens on the basement membrane of different tissues, the renal disfunction as encountered in burn patients might partly be explained on the basis of cross reacting antibodies. However, none of the sera tested showed a positive reaction in the passive haemagglutination test using glomerular basement membrane of human kidney as antigen.

With indirect immunofluorescence techniques using guinea-pig oral mucosa as substrate, no antibodies against basement membrane could be detected either.

4. Routine determination (7) of antibodies against the following antigens, which are known to appear in by now well established auto-immune disease, were negative against the antigen substrate of gastric mucosa, salivary gland, thyroid gland, skeletal muscle, smooth muscle and mitochondria.

5. As whole skin contains serumproteins, the appearance of antiglobulins after thermal injury is feasible. Indeed Kano (11) and Quismorio (19) et al. demonstrated the appearance of a rheumatoid factor using the latex fixation test. However, in our study we were unable with the more reliable Waaler-Rose test to demonstrate an antiglobulin. With a more sensitive haemagglutination technique which is routinely used in our laboratory for the typing of various immunoglobulin classes and subclasses, positive reactions were detected in three patients only: In the serum of a 5 year old boy an antiglobulin was found which was directed against Gm(Pa), which is a recently discovered (15) Gm-allotype of the IgG-3. As the boy showed this Gm(Pa)-allotype himself and the antibody was not present in his serum 3 days after the accident, and as he did not receive whole blood transfusions, it is most likely that we are dealing with a true auto-antibody. In 2 other patients the antiglobulins were specifically directed against IgG-1 and IgG-2 respectively. A peculiarity of these antibodies is the fact that the haemagglutination could not be blocked by preincubation of the sera with the corresponding antigen in native form, but only when the antigen was bound to erythrocytes. This fact indicates that these antibodies are so-called anti-antibodies, as described by Milgrom (16) in 1956. The significance of these anti-antibodies, which are also seen after organ transplantation in man (12, 22), remains speculative. Possibly they enhance the removal of foreign or denatured proteins from the circulation.

6. Since skin is the first organ to be inflicted in burn injury, the appearance of antibo-

dies directed against skin is most likely. With the indirect immunofluorescence technique on guinea-pig oral mucosa we were able to detect anti-skin antibodies in 8 out of 23 patients. As also reported by others (19, 20, 21) we noticed the pemphigus-like pattern as displayed by these antibodies. Most antibodies were seen 2 weeks after the injury and belonged to the various immunoglobulin classes, especially IgG.

From 4 patients biopsies of normal unafflicted skin were taken two weeks after the injury as well. In two cases biopsies revealed staining for IgA which was localized intercellularly. Elution experiments on the skin sections from one of these patients did not

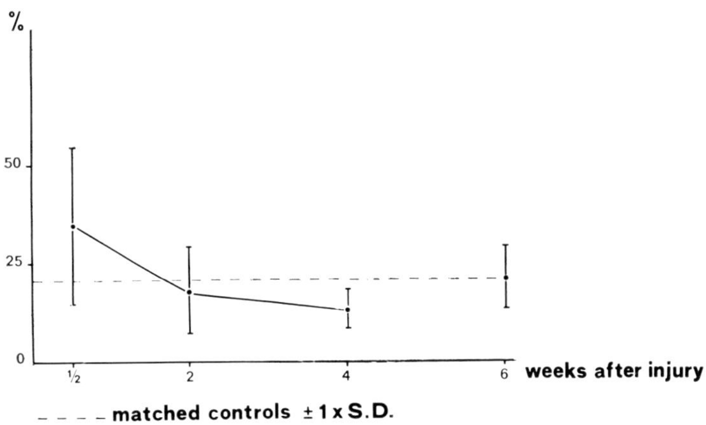

Fig. 1. Proportion of complement-reactive lymphocytes in five burned patients (±1 × S.D.)

recover these antibodies. The serum from the other patient showed circulating IgA-antibodies against an intercellular substance of the epithelial of two unrelated and healthy individuals. The significance of the anti-skin antibodies remains doubtfull. We could not establish an apparent correlation between the incidence of these antibodies and the extent of the burn injury or the clinical outcome (survival). There was no relation between the incidence of these antibodies and any form of therapy such as early or late necrectomy. The appearance of an infection by a particular micro-organism did not have any effect on these antibodies. As mentioned earlier similar antibodies are also found obligatorily in the clinical entity of pemphigus vulgaris (2). However, we did not observe the appearance of any skin affliction in our patients in otherwise unharmed areas.

Possibly the circulating skin-antibodies can be regarded as a subclinical form of pemphigus vulgaris. In this respect it is note-worthy to mention that Beutner (3) and colleagues described a burn patient with circulating pemphigus-like antibodies who developed pemphigus foliaceus.

In regard to the pathophysiology of auto-immunity in burn patients our studies (14) on the cellular immune status seem to be of particular interest. It could be shown that the function of the thymus-dependent lymphocyte population *in vitro* as measured in the mixed lymphocyte culture technique is significantly impaired during a two-week period post burn, when compared with adequate controls. Fig. 1 shows, however, that during the same period the proportion of bone marrow derived lymphocytes in the peripheral blood from burn patients is found to be significantly increased, as measured by the proportion of complement-reactive-lymphocytes, which has been described to be a parameter of the B-cells present (4).

Conclusion

In view of the results on cellular immunity the inducement of autoimmune phenomena might be ascribed to a temporarily increased B-cell population. It has been postulated by Allison et al. (1) that auto-antibodies may also appear due to an impairment of T-cells which normally regulate the immune tolerance of the organism. As a subsequent result of lack of control by the T-cell a highly functional and possibly uncontrolled B-cell population arises after burn injury, which may produce auto-antibodies either spontaneously or in response to altered auto-antigens.

In summary it can be concluded that according to this study the appearance of autoimmune phenomena after thermal injury are rather exceptional and so far no correlation with clinical parameters could be established.

References

1. Allison, A. C., Denman, A. M. and Barnes, R. D. (1971): Cooperating and controlling functions of thymus-derived lymphocytes in relation to autoimmunity. Lancet 2 : 135.
2. Beutner, E. H. (1969): Autoimmunity in pemphigus and pemphigoid. In: Textbook of Immunopathology. Vol II. Eds. P. A. Miescher; H. J. Müller-Eberhard, 655.
3. Beutner, E. H. (1969): The diagnosis of pemphigus. Brit. J. Derm. 84 : 594.
4. Bianco, C., Patrick, R. and Nussenzweig, V. (1970): A population of lymphocytes bearing a membrane receptor for antigen-antibody-complement complexes. I. Separation and characterization. J. exp. Med. 132 : 702.
5. Bray, J. P., Estess, F. and Bass, J. A. (1969): Anticollagen antibodies following thermal trauma. Proc. Soc. exp. Biol. Med. 130 : 394.
6. Dygin, V. P. and Kliachkin, L. M. (1965): Autoimmune hemolytic anemia in burn sickness. Problemy Gematologii 10 : 37.
7. Feltkamp, T. E. W. and Rossum, A. L. van (1968): Antibodies to salivary duct cells, and other auto-antibodies, in patients with Sjögren's syndrome and other idiopathic autoimmune diseases. Clin. exp. Imm. 3 : 1.
8. Fisher, J. P. (1965): Soluble substances of human stratum corneum. J. invest. Derm. 44 : 43.
9. Holder, I. A. and Jogan, M. (1970): Antigenic components of normal and burned mouse skin. Experientia 25 : 1363.
10. Hutchinson, R., Patel, R. and MacArthur, J. (1971): Rheumatoid, antinuclear and antileukocyte cytotoxic factors in patients with burns. Amer. J. Surg. 122 : 520.
11. Kano, K., Milgrom, F. and Rapaport, F. T. (1967): Immunologic studies in thermal injury: heterophile antibodies. Proc. Soc. exp. Biol. Med. 125 : 142.
12. Kano, K. and Milgrom, F. (1968): Anti-gamma-globulin factors in human allograft recipients. Transpl. 6 : 111.
13. Kolker, I. I. (1965): Immunopathological data on pathogenesis of burn disease and glomerulonephritis. Fed. Proc. 24 : T 507.
14. Leguit, Jr., P., Meinesz, A., Zeijlemaker, W. P., Schellekens, P. Th. A. and Eijsvoogel, V. P. (1973): Immunological studies in burn patients. I-Lymphocyte transformation in vitro. Clin. exp. Immun. 44 : 101.
15. Loghem, E. van and Grobbelaar, B. G. (1971): A new genetic marker of human IgG3 immunoglobulins. Vox Sang. 21 : 405.
16. Milgrom, F., Dubiski, S. and Wozniczko, G. (1956): Human sera with "anti-antibody" Vox Sang. 1 : 172.
17. Pavkova, L. (1962): Formation and significance of auto-antibodies in burned patients. Vox Sang. 7 : 116.
18. Price, W. R., Wood, M. and Childers, D. (1969): Presence of leukocyte antibodies in major thermal burns. Amer. J. Surg. 118 : 871.
19. Quismorio, F. P., Bland, S. L. and Friou, G. J. (1971): Auto-immunity in thermal injury: occurrence of rheumatoid factors, antinuclear antibodies and anti-epithelial antibodies. Clin. exp. Imm. 8 : 701.
20. Thivolet, J. and Beyvin, A. J. (1968): Recherche par immunofluorescence d'autoanticorps sériques vis-à-vis des constituants de l'epiderme chez les brûlés. Experientia (Basel). 24 : 945.

21. TRIFTSHAUSER, C., WYPICH, J., CLOUTIER, L. C. and BEUTNER, E. H. (1971): Fluorescent antibody studies of pemphigus-like antibodies in burn sera. Ann. N.Y. Acad. Sci. 177 : 227.
22. WALLER, M., IRBY, R., MULLINAX, F. and TOONE, JR., E. C. (1965): Connective-tissue disease and rheumatoid factors in patients with renal transplants. New Eng. J. Med. 273 : 12.

P. L., Chirurgische Kliniek,
Binnengasthuis,
Amsterdam, The Netherlands

COMPLEMENT AND ACUTE BURN TRAUMA

S. B. DAY, J. EELKEMA, R. A. GOOD and N. K. DAY

Departments of Pathology, Laboratory Medicine and Research Surgery, University of Minnesota Medical School, Minneapolis, 55455, U.S.A.

We have pointed out in preceding studies (2, 3) the desirability that acute severe burn trauma be viewed as a *total body injury* rather than as the infliction of a cutaneous insult followed by "complications." Our present studies are concerned with the complement (C) system.

Complement, an important immunological amplification complex in the body, appears closely related to two "total body systems" of importance to the burn surgeon — the Kinin system and mechanisms of clotting. Generally speaking few studies have explored relationships between perturbations of the C system and acute severe burn injury.

We now report observations for time sequence studies in which complement active serum proteins, considered of importance in certain expressions of immunity, have been examined before and immediately following acute burn injury in experiments upon homiothermic and poikilothermic animals. Observations are presented for serum complement components C1, C2, C3, C4, C5, C8, and C9.

Materials and Methods

250 g adult Sprague Dawley rats were used in all homiothermic studies. The American Bullfrog (Rana Catesbeiana) was used in the poikilothermic experiments. All animals were bled prior to thermal injury and afterwards at sequential intervals of 6, 20, 68, 120, hours and up to a week post trauma. Blood was drawn by cardiac puncture and allowed to clot for one hour at room temperature, centrifuged, and the sera preserved at −70 degrees of centigrade until ready for use.

Standard full thickness burns, approximately 25 per cent total body surface, were produced on the backs of lightly anesthetised animals with the use of a standard restraining apparatus. Burn injury was provoked by immersion of the selected skin area in water heated to 99 ± 1 degrees of centigrade for 20 seconds. Total proteins were estimated

* This study was supported in part by a Grant in Aid from the Minnesota Medical Foundation.— Dr. Stacey B. Day is Conservator and Head, Bell Museum of Pathobiology and Associate Professor, Laboratory Medicine and Pathology, University of Minnesota Medical School.

with the use of the method of Folin and Ciocalten (4). Assays of total hemolytic complement CH50 and of the C components Cl to C9 were carried out by the method of Geiger and associates (5).

Results

Total hemolytic C dropped within six hours in the warm blooded animals (35.4 per cent of normal value) and remained depressed until 20 hours post burn. After this time, the total CH50 increased quite rapidly and reached normal values within 120 hours. In contrast, although the total protein showed an initial decrease, its level did not fluctuate greatly up to at least 100 hours.

Repeat experimental studies confirmed this pattern of events. C titer, after an initial fall, returned to normal values within 60–80 hours (three to four days), whereas the total protein was still depressed at that time. In a study of eight female adrenalectomised rats and in 17 day pregnant rats, the pattern of CH50 and protein change was similar to that reported above. *When individual C components were assayed after burn trauma, it was shown that C1, C4, C3, and C8 levels were reduced but C9 was elevated.*

With respect to studies in the poikilothermic animals (frogs), an initial increase in total hemolytic complement (21 per cent) was followed by a severe drop at 25 hours post burn injury. After 48–72 hours post burn a gradual increase in CH50 values occurred. When protein values were determined, no significant changes could be observed. These experiments in fact tend to yield results that appear to be similar to those described for the homiothermic animals.

Discussion

Studies of serum complement show that total hemolytic complement actively drops sharply to lowest levels within six hours after the burn and then begins a return toward normal levels within the succeeding hours. Normal and even higher than normal levels are reached 60 to 100 hours after the burn. Analysis of the complement components shows that levels of each of the first individual components parallel in their drop and rise the total hemolytic complement levels after a burn. However, levels of C9 are sharply dissociated from the others. From a few after the burn, C9 shows significant elevations over the normal level. The decline of complement and complement components in the blood are parallel to the decline of total serum proteins. However, recovery of the C levels after the burn reveals striking dissociation of both total complement and individual complement components from the total serum protein levels. Prior studies, especially in man, have revealed the early drop of serum complement soon after a burn with recovery to normal and in some instances to higher than normal levels within four to seven days (1). The basis for the rapid return to normal or elevated C and C component levels can be fully explained only by further study. In considering the basis for the rapid loss of C and early C components from serum, Arturson and Fjellstrom postulated activation of the complement system by antibodies directed against burned skin (1). To us, however, the parallel of losses or drop of C and C component levels to known losses and drop of serum levels of other serum proteins suggests that immunologic explanations of these dramatic changes in C serum levels may require no immunologic explanation. Losses into the burn site and from permeable vessels could be explanation enough.

The maximal susceptibility of burned animals and of burned patients to infection coincides temporally with the maximum drop in serum complement and C components and could indeed be explained in part at least by these changes. Our observations one adrenalectomised animals suggest to us adrenal steroid release associated with stress may also be responsible in part for the overall biologic perspective demonstrated in these investigations. In our studies, C9 did not behave like either the total serum proteins, total complement or other C components. The basis for the dissociation of C9 from the other complement components after burns is not clear but is consonent with other studies which show a sharp dissociation of C9 and other complement components when viewed from the perspective of the molecular relationships (6).

With respect to our finding in the poikilothermic studies, our results do not appear to be disimilar nor warrant an explanation different to that postulated above. Full explanation of such interesting dissociations as we have described must await further understanding in comparison of total serum proteins and other acute phase reactants following experimental acute burn trauma and analysis.

References

1. Arturson, A. and Fjellstrom, K. E. (1963): Alterations of serum complement factors following Burn Trauma. Transactions Third International Congress on Plastic Surgery, Washington D.C., 99.
2. Day, S. B., MacMillan, B. G. and Altemeier, W. A. (1972): Curling's Ulcer: An Experiment of Nature. Springfield, III., Charles C. Thomas Publisher.
3. Day, S. B. (1973): Trauma and Trauma Emergent Problems. St. Louis, Mo. Warren H. Green Publ.
4. Folin, O. and Ciocalten, V. (1927): On tyrosine and tryptophane determinations in proteins. J. Biol. 73 : 627.
5. Geiger, H., Day, N. K. and Good, R. A.: Methods for the measurement of nine components of hemolytic complement in rat serum. (In preparation).
6. Kolb, W. K., Maxby, J. A., Arroyave, C. M. and Mulier - Eberhard, H. J. (1972): Molecular analysis of the membrane attack mechanism of complement. J. exp. Med. 135 : 549.

S. B. D., Bell Museum of Pathology,
198 Jackson Hall,
Minneapolis, Minnesota 55455, U.S.A.

THE EPIDEMIOLOGY OF BURN WOUND SEPSIS IN AN INTENSIVE CARE UNIT

B. G. MacMILLAN and M. P. MALEY

Shriners Burns Institute, Cincinnati Unit — Cincinnati, Ohio, U.S.A.

Introduction

A comprehensive bacteriological study of patients and their environment in the intensive care unit of the Shriners Cincinnati Burn Unit has been carried out during the past five years. The Cincinnati Unit was designed to study optimal use of conventional air handling and reverse isolation techniques for the control of infections in burn patients. Since it has been in operation, the influence of these measures on the incidence of infections in burn patients has been under evaluation.

Material and Methods

One half of the patients treated in the unit have been colonized with *Pseudomonas aeruginosa* at some time during their hospitalization. All cultures of Pseudomonas were serotyped on the basis of major typing reactions. Serotype 2 was the most prevalent in cultures from patients with fatal burn wound sepsis, and serotype 1 was the most common in nonfatal Pseudomonas infections. Eighty-three percent of the cultures from burn patients and their environment could be identified by serotyping and 91 per cent by phage typing. Pyocine typing was used as an adjunct to the other two methods.

During a three-month period, 285 cultures of *Pseudomonas aeruginosa* were isolated from patients. Thirty-one patients were admitted to the hospital during this period and 16 of these patients acquired positive cultures for Pseudomonas while hospitalized. Three patients had positive cultures for *Pseudomonas aeruginosa* upon admission, and 13 patients acquired their *Pseudomonas aeruginosa* organism during their hospital stay. The average period of hospitalization prior to acquiring a *Pseudomonas aeruginosa* infection was 9.9 days. During the same three-month period, 255 *Pseudomonas aeruginosa* cultures were isolated from non-patient sources. Air cultures obtained by sediment plates, the TDL slit sampler and the Anderson sampler, as well as nebulizers, counter surfaces and nurses' hands were constantly negative during the entire period. Bed rails were positive for *Pseudomonas* approximately one half of the times cultured. The two major sources of environmental contamination in this intensive care unit were the sinks and the hydrotherapy equipment. While sink drains were the highest source of contamination and were positive in essentially 100 per cent of all cultures, positive cultures from sink basins were obtained in only 20 per cent of these studies. The faucet cultures were constantly negative, but in subsequent studies have been found to be positive in high usage areas.

Discussion

The measures for the control of infection in burn patients consisted of the use of specific topical antibacterial agents, the use of allografts, xenografts and synthetic skin substitutes, reinforcing the patient's immune response by active and passive immunization measures, nutritional support by oral hyperalimentation, and the early closure of the burn wounds with aggressive debridement or excision and coverage with expanded autogenous tissue.

The measures for the control of *Pseudomonas aeruginosa* in the environment of the patient consisted of the use of masks, gloves, caps, gowns and hand washing after each treatment for personnel, the decontamination of faucets and traps with 10 per cent formalin, and frequent cleansing of basins with abrasive cleansers, as well as the use of 2 per cent Ves-Phene for the sterilization of sinks. All mops were sterilized with 2 per cent Ves-Phene three times a day prior to mopping of the floors. To minimize contamination from food sources, dry storage was utilized and cooking done when possible. Daily cleansing of storage units in the patient care unit, periodic culturing of soap dishes and containers, and gas or cold sterilization of respiratory equipment used on patients. Sterility of temperature control units was maintained by the circulation of 2 per cent phenol, and plastic liners were used in conjunction with hydrotherapy equipment after the removal of agitators and traps to prevent cross contamination from these sources.

These environmental control measures used in the Cincinnati Unit of the Shriners Burns Institute have shown that sophisticated laminar flow units for environmental control are not necessary, and that rather simple modifications of established routines and adherence to strict reverse isolation techniques can contain the patient's own bacteria to his environment and prevent cross contamination within the unit. Serotyping techniques have shown that 3 or 4 patients can be treated in the same intensive care unit without disseminating their organisms to other patients while being cared for in these facilities.

All of these measures have been carried out voluntarily by personnel in the unit with the assistance of color coding. The patient care unit is isolated from the remainder of the medical center environment by outside observation corridors, and attire is completely changed by all personnel entering the unit. Transfer areas prevent the free movement of equipment and supplies in and out of the area without proper cleansing and inspection.

This concept of patient care has made it possible to reduce the ambient bacterial flora in the unit by approximately two thirds. However, the same qualitative distribution exists in this unit as exists in the adult burn unit of the Cincinnati General Hospital.

Since the Shriners Cincinnati Burn Unit has been in operation, the mortality rate has progressively fallen from a high of 30 per cent in 1967 to a low of 4 per cent in 1972. Septic deaths during this period have accounted for 40 per cent of the deaths occurring within the unit. *Pseudomonas aeruginosa* has been responsible for 36 per cent of these deaths, and *Staphylococcus aureus*, *Klebsiella*, *Paracolobactrum*, *E. coli*, *Enterobacter* and *Candida albicans* for 3, 1, 1, 1, 1, and 12 per cent, respectively. Pulmonary deaths have accounted for 26 per cent of the mortalities, and cardiovascular and gastrointestinal for 10 and 3 per cent, respectively. Since 1964, the surface area associated with a 50 per cent mortality rate has increased from 35 to 75 per cent of the total body surface.

This experience has shown that rigid adherence to strict reverse isolation techniques, combined with optimal local and systemic supportive measures, at this time can give the patient the best chance for survival.

B. G. MacM., 202 Goodman St.,
Cincinnati, Ohio 45219, U.S.A.

PATTERNS OF BURN WOUND SEPSIS DURING THE PAST 30 YEARS

B. G. MacMILLAN

Shriners Burns Institute, Cincinnati Unit, Cincinnati, Ohio, U.S.A.

Introduction

The patterns of burn wound sepsis since 1942, as experienced in the burn units of the Cincinnati General Hospital and the Shriners Cincinnati Burns Institute, have been reviewed. During this period, the pattern of burn wound sepsis has changed from gram-positive organisms to gram-negative organisms to fungal organisms and, recently, to viral pathogens. To determine the influence of supportive measures and environmental control on the survival of burn patients, this study has been undertaken.

Material and Methods

In this 30-year period, four groups of patients have been studied, the first between 1942 and 1944, consisting of 147 patients treated with sulfonamides, the second between 1951 and 1953, consisting of 318 patients treated with penicillin and broad-spectrum antibiotics the third between 1957 and 1960, consisting of 392 patients treated with specific anti-staphylococcal antibiotics, and the fourth group between 1965 and 1972, consisting of 552 patients, 356 of whom were treated with topical antibacterial agents, 170 with systemic gentamicin, 184 with heptavalent vaccine, 23 with *Pseudomonas* hyperimmune globulin, 12 with amphotericin, 58 with excisional therapy and 91 with allografts and 132 with xenografts.

Discussion

The incidence of septicemia during these four periods has fallen from a high of 50 per cent in Group I to an incidence of 20 per cent in Group IV. The significant improvement in mortality has occurred in Group IV, where the mortality rates for 1964 to 1972 were 20, 15, 26, 30, 11, 14, 11, 29 and 4 per cent respectively. The overall mortality rate for this period was 12 per cent. Septicemia was the cause of death in 36 per cent of these patients, with pulmonary complications accounting for 18 per cent, cardiovascular complications for 7 per cent, gastrointestinal complications for 2 per cent, and other complications for 3 per cent. The organisms most commonly involved in septic complications were the

Pseudomonas aeruginosa, *Staphylococcus aureus*, *Klebsiella*, *Paracolobactrum*, *Escherichia coli*, *Enterobacter*, and *Candida albicans*.

The group of 356 patients treated with topical antibacterial agents consisted of 85 patients treated with Sulfamylon, 25 with silver nitrate, 67 with silver sulfadiazine and 179 with gentamicin. When the LA-50 for these agents is plotted by linear regression, the respective surface areas for Sulfamylon, silver nitrate, silver sulfadiazine and gentamicin were found to be 46, 52, 60 and 63 per cent, respectively. For this reason, gentamicin, in the form of either ointment or cream, has been used routinely in those patients in whom invasive burn wound sepsis threatens survival.

Systemic gentamicin has also been found to have a beneficial effect on invasive burn wound sepsis. When the LA-50 survivals for patients treated systemically with gentamicin between the years of 1967 and 1972 are plotted, the associated surface areas have been noted to increase from 40 per cent in 1967 to 75 per cent in 1972.

Immunological support has also been of great benefit. In the group of 184 patients treated with the Fisher heptavalent vaccine between 1968 and 1972, 5 patients or 3 per cent died as a result of *Pseudomonas aeruginosa* sepsis. This was in contrast to a 15 per cent mortality rate in the control series of 75 patients. In a group of 13 burn patients treated with *Pseudomonas* hyperimmune serum, representing a group of patients who could not be actively immunized prior to the fifth postburn day, only 2 deaths occurred.

Amphotericin has been used systemically in a group of 12 patients for invasive *Candida albicans* septicemia. Six patients responded to a ten-day course of therapy and survived.

The mortality rate in a group of 58 children recently treated with early excision has been found to be 5 per cent. Burn wounds were excised between the third and the 24th postburn day, were totally closed with autografts immediately by expansion techniques when possible, and when sufficient autogenous tissue was not available, closure was completed with allografts and xenografts. The morbidity and mortality in this group of patients was improved.

This study indicates that all of these measures have been effective in containing burn wound sepsis and in improving survival. The significant determinants for this improvement in survival can be related to the control of the patient's environment, intensive supportive care in special care facilities, aggressive nutritional support, reinforcement of the patient's immune response by active and passive immunization, and early closure of the burn wound by either aggressive debridement or excision, followed by total autogenous coverage or, if this is not possible, complemented with allograft and xenograft coverage. The LA-50 mortality rate reflected in the 552 patients treated in the fourth group substantiates this conclusion. The LA-50 in the beginning of this period was 35 per cent, and this has steadily increased to a total body surface burn of 75 per cent, which is now associated with a 50 per cent mortality rate.

B.G.MacM., 202 Goodman St.,
Cincinnati, Ohio 45219, U.S.A.

TABLES AIDING DIFFERENTIAL DIAGNOSIS OF BURN SEPSIS

S. A. POLISHCHUK

V. M. Bogoslavskii Hospital Surgical Clinic, A. M. Gorkii State Medical Institute, Donetsk, U.S.S.R.

The diagnostics of burn sepsis has still remained difficult owing to the lack of pathognomic symptoms characteristic of this state. The situation is further complicated by the lack of a consensus of opinions concerning the interpretation of the term "burn sepsis". The introduction of the term "burn wound sepsis" has widened the gap dividing the viewpoints of combustologists in different countries. In our opinion, it is convenient to use the term "burn sepsis" for generalized sepsis in victims of burn, and to consider this disease a complication of the burn disease as a whole, not only of the wound process alone. As in any sepsis, two meaningful clinical forms of burn sepsis may be distinguished, namely, burn septicaemia and burn septicopyaemia, according to the absence or presence of metastases of purulent infection. A unification of terms would facilitate mutual understanding among combustologists in different countries.

Postmortal diagnostics of burn sepsis is merely of academic significance; the diagnosis should be established as early as possible. Every combustologist, however, knows how difficult a severe burn disease is to differentiate from burn sepsis. The endeavour aimed at facilitating the diagnostics of burn sepsis is justifiable and of essential importance. These considerations prompted us to elaborate tables for differential diagnosis of burn sepsis. We chose the method of linear discriminant functions, which belongs to the most widely used methods for pattern recognition inclusive of pathological processes. In this way the adjoined Tables 1 and 2 were produced.

Electronic-computer analyses were made of 187 observations including 47 symptoms. Thirty-one symptoms were found essential for differential diagnostics, and included in the tables. Table 1 is based on comparative investigations of a group of 142 patients with proved burn sepsis and a group of 36 patients in whom clinical examinations led to suspicion of sepsis which, however, was disproved by necropsy. Each of the two groups is large enough to allow the findings to be considered representative. Table 2 is based on a comparison (using the same method) of 70 patients with burn septicopyaemia with 72 patients with burn septicaemia.

The following characteristics were found meaningless for the differential diagnosis: the patient's age, blood group (ABO system), Rh type, and counts of nonsegmented and segmented neutrophils in the differential leukocyte count. On the other hand, the fol-

TABLE 1

Burn sepsis present or absent?

No.	Symptom	Range of values	Diagn. index
1	Burnt area, total	under 20 per cent 20–50 per cent over 50 per cent	0 5 10
2	Area of deep burns	under 10 per cent 10–20 per cent over 20 per cent	0 2 7
3	Burn of airways	present absent	3 0
4	Burn shock, moderate severity	present absent	1 0
5	Burn shock, medium severity	present absent	2 0
6	Burn shock, severe	present absent	3 0
7	Chill	present absent	6 0
8	Hyperhidrosis	present absent	5 0
9	Mental disturbances (delirium)	present absent	–2 0
10	Abdominal swelling	present absent	1 0
11	Oliguria	present absent	7 0
12	Anuria	present absent	–9 0
13	Dyspnoe	present absent	9 0
14	Tachycardia	present absent	9 0
15	Hypotension	present absent	–2 0
16	Pneumonia	present absent	3 0
17	Temperature fluctuation	by less than 1 degree of centigrade by 1–2 degrees of centigrade by more than 2 degrees of centigrade	0 2 5
18	Leukocyte count, thous/mm^3 of blood	under 10 10–20 over 20	0 1 3

TABLE 2

Septicaemia or septicopyaemia?

No.	Symptom	Range of values	Diagn. index
1	Burnt area, total	under 20 per cent 20–50 per cent over 50 per cent	0 –4 –8
2	Area of deep burns	under 10 per cent 10–20 per cent over 20 per cent	0 –2 –4
3	Burn of airways	present absent	–3 0
4	Burn shock, moderate severity	present absent	3 0
5	Burn shock, medium severity	present absent	2 0
6	Burn shock, severe	present absent	–4 0
7	Chill	present absent	8 0
8	Hyperhidrosis	present absent	8 0
9	Mental disturbances (delirium)	present absent	2 0
10	Abdominal swelling	present absent	3 0
11	Oliguria	present absent	4 0
12	Anuria	present absent	–9 0
13	Dyspnoe	present absent	1 0
14	Tachycardia	present absent	–1 0
15	Hypotension	present absent	–2 0
16	Pneumonia	present absent	–5 0
17	Temperature fluctuation	by less than 1 degree of centigrade 1–2 degres of centigrade more than 2 degrees of centigrade	0 2 4
18	Leukocyte count, thous./mm^3 of blood	under 10 10–20 over 20	0 2 4

Table 1 continued

No.	Symptom	Range of values	Diagn. index
19	Promyelocytes	present absent	−2 0
20	Myelocytes	present absent	1 0
21	Juvenile neutrophils	present absent	1 0
22	Bilirubin level in serum, mg/100 ml	under 1 1–2 over 2	0 1 2
23	Transitory bacteriaemia	present absent	3 0
24	Intensive bacteriaemia	present absent	9 0
25	Skin petechiae	present absent	8 0
26	Decubitus	present absent	6 0
27	Dry gangraene of wound	present absent	−3 0
28	Moist gangraene of wound	present absent	9 0
29	Secondary/tertiary necrosis	present absent	9 0
30	Purulent phlegmons	present absent	7 0
31	Arthritis	absent 1 joint 2 and more joints	0 1 2

When analyzing the given case, obtain the *algebraic sum* of diagnostic indexes.
If the sum is
less than 30: sepsis is probably not present;
greater than 30, but less than 48: no univocal diagnosis is possible;
greater than 48: burn sepsis is probably present.

Table 2 continued

No.	Symptom	Range of values	Diagn. index
19	Promyelocytes	present absent	−2 0
20	Myelocytes	present absent	1 0
21	Juvenile neutrophils	present absent	1 0
22	Bilirubin level in serum, mg/100 ml	under 1 1–2 over 2	0 1 2
23	Transitory bacteriaemia	present absent	−3 0
24	Intensive bacteriaemia	present absent	−4 0
25	Skin petechiae	present absent	−7 0
26	Decubitus	present absent	−4 0
27	Dry gangraene of wound	present absent	−2 0
28	Moist gangraene of wound	present absent	−4 0
29	Secondary/tertiary necrosis	present absent	−7 0
30	Purulent phlegmons	present absent	−6 0
31	Arthritis	absent 1 joint 2 and more joints	0 1 2

When analyzing the given case, obtain the *algebraic sum* of diagnostic indexes.
If the sum is
less than −28: septicaemia is probably present; greater than −28, but less than −10: no univocal diagnosis is possible;
greater than −10: septicopyaemia is apparently present.

lowing characteristics were found meaningful for the diagnosis of sepsis: counts of promyelocytes, myelocytes, and juvenile forms. Meaningless was found the presence or absence of icterus, and meaningful, the serum bilirubin level. Also meaningless was the presence or absence of osteomyelitis, whereas the presence of arthritis, and even the number of joints afflicted by arthritis, were found to be meaningful symptoms.

The use of the tables is easy. If the physician suspects that the burn disease is complicated by sepsis, he uses the table for finding the algebraic sum of the diagnostic indexes applicable to his patient. If the sum is less than +30, there is a high probability that the burn disease, even if severe, is *not accompanied by burn sepsis*. If the sum is greater than +30, but less than +48, no univocal diagnosis is possible, and observation must be continued. If the sum is greater than +48, *burn sepsis* may be accepted to be *present*. In such an instance, all therapeutic means available are intensified; the authors ascribe great importance to direct blood transfusions. An established presence of burn sepsis may justify even extreme measures of treatment, for example, amputation.

If the diagnosis of sepsis is established beyond any doubt in general, then Table 2 may be used to advantage for differentiating the forms of burn sepsis, namely, septicaemia or septicopyaemia. The algebraic sum (respecting the plus or minus signs) of diagnostic indexes is obtained from the table. If the sum is less than —28, septicaemia is probably present. If the sum is greater than —28, but less than —10, no univocal diagnosis is possible. If the sum is greater than —10, septicopyaemia may be accepted to be present, even if no metastases of purulent infection are manifest.

In conclusion, several circumstances have to be pointed out. Certain symptoms were not included in the tables, which, although clinically evaluable and of indubitable import, are difficult to express in numerical values. Any clinician, no doubt, acknowledges the importance of symptoms of sepsis such as wound purulence after venesection, lysis of epithelium recently formed on almost healed segments of burnt skin, lysis of transplanted and almost healed autologous skin patches, and similar ones. Furthermore, the diagnostic importance of any striking discrepancy between the character and extent of the lesion on the one hand, and the severity of the patient's state on the other hand, has been established years ago. All of such symptoms are the basis of the physician's suspicion of burn sepsis. No tables can surrogate medical thinking. The essential purpose of our or other tables is to facilitate a comprehensive appraisal of various phenomena, that is to say, to aid and not to replace thinking. If our tables help draw the combustologist's attention to a potential presence of burn sepsis and instigate his use of all — even extreme — therapeutic means for saving the life of a burn victim, then the endeavour spent in their accomplishment was not in vain.

S. A. P., Surgical Clinic,
V. M. Bogosloavskii Hospital,
Donetsk, U.S.S.R.

THERAPY OF BURNS IN CHILDREN

V. TOŠOVSKÝ, B. APETAUROVÁ, B. FIŠER and M. HRUBANTOVÁ

Clinic of Paediatric Surgery, Paediatric Faculty Hospital, Prague, Czechoslovakia

The main problem is how to prevent or how to combat the microbial infection already present, endangering the patient's life and often causing his death.

The virulence and growth of bacteria depend on various factors (shock, dehydration, thermal injury of skin, antibiotics, etc.). Preventive administration of antibiotics or their use according to the cultivation and sensitivity carries with it the danger of producing resistant bacterial strains. Staphylococcus albus, Staphylococcus epidermidis and Staphylococcus pyogenes aureus are not so dangerous as Pseudomonas aeruginosa and Proteus vulgaris.

However, this communication does not concentrate on aspects of immunology and bacteriology.

In this paper, we should like to discuss the method of local antibacterial therapy for burns which has been successfully used at our department over the past three years.

We are well aware of the fact that the prevalent trend in contemporary treatment of burns is the open method with early necrectomy and transplantation. However, in burned children we observe often well preserved islands of skin from which the regeneration of the skin takes place. We believe these cases to be suitable for treatment with Fox's silver-sulfathiazol ointment. Since 1970 we have been treating 88 burned children up to the age of 3 years. We do not use the compressive dressing any longer. We should like to stress the difference between Fox's ointment and the silver nitrate which was used in the past. Fox utilizes the oligodynamic effect of silver and the bactericidal effect of sulfonamides. Therefore, it is not a mixture of two compounds, but the synthesis of a new matter free of the irritating effect of silver nitrate and the sensitising effect of sulfonamides. Silver sulfathiazol is not blocked by para-amino-benzoic acid as is the case in pure sulfonamides.

Silversulfathiazol is affecting cells of Pseudomonas aeruginosa in such a way that these bind silver while sulfathiazol remains freely effective on their surface. This effect is supported by ribonucleic and desoxiribonucleic acid. The result of this treatment was dependent upon the time elapsed between the injury and commencement of the therapy.

During the first two years the majority of patients were those previously treated in other hospitals by dressings and suffering from sepsis. Only in the last year are most of the patients delivered to our hospital shortly after injury.

We should like to demonstrate only one patient from each group.

Case 1. A three-year old girl treated for two weeks by compressive dressings for scalds of the 2nd and 3rd degree involving cca 70 p. c. BSA. Admitted in severe sepsis. The treatment was very difficult. An unusual complication was a luxation of the hip, which had to be reduced by operation.

Case 2. This girl with severe scalds was treated from the beginning by silver-sulfathiazol ointment. The healing was uneventful.

Fox pointed out the importance of small islands of epithelium which are present even in deep burns. Presuming that we are able to prevent infection, epithelisation from these islands is very quick.

We treated 88 patients. In 21 patients transferred to our department on the 7th–14th day after injury Staphylococcus pyogenes was present. This infection was eradicated successfully by silver-sulfathiazol ointment in 7–14 days.

In 2 patients treated previously by dressing Pseudomonas infection was present. This was eradicated after 10 days of silver-sulfathiazol therapy.

In 3 patients mixed infection was present (E. coli, Aerobacter, Proteus, Candida albicans). On the 12th day of treatment the swabs were negative.

In 62 children admitted shortly after injury and treated by Fox's ointment the swabs were negative. We lost three children for severe sepsis.

Concluding our experiences with silver-sulfathiazol ointment we can say that it proved to be very effective. Moreover, we used this therapy successfully in extensive infected wounds of other ethiology.

Mortality has decreased considerably and the time of treatment shortened by more than one half.

V. T., Clinic of Paediatric Surgery,
Ke Karlovu 2,
121 09 Praha 2, Czechoslovakia

WARM AIR TREATMENT OF BURNS IN THE STERAIR UNIT

T. MIDTVEDT and O. M. UGLAND

Burns Unit, Department of Surgery, and Bacteriological Unit, Department of Clinical Chemistry, University Hospital of Oslo, Akershus, Norway

Isolation in a clean ward room has for many years been considered an indispensible requisite in the treatment of burns. More recently some groups, especially the Birke — Liljedahl group in Stockholm, called attention to the large caloric losses in patients with extensive burns — an observation which prompted the development of the warm air treatment. Hoping to gain profit from a combination of these two principles in an easy way, we have tested a modified Pathfinder STERAIR unit in treating severe burns in our department (Fig. 1).

Essentially, the STERAIR unit envelops the patient's bed in sterile air, within an enclosing "air curtain". A console, standing behind the head of a normal hospital bed, contains the STERAIR Fan/Filter system. A continuously-rated fan unit draws in air, through dual pre-filters near the base of the console and delivers it through an absolute filter at the top. Free from bacteria, the air is discharged through openings in the underside of a canopy which projects from the console, over the bed. A main flow, at imperceptibly low velocity, sweeps downward over the whole area of the bed. A carefully directed flow, at higher velocity, emerges from the periphery of the canopy to form the "air curtain" within which the main flow is confined. Though there is no sensation of draught over the area of the bed, the peripheral curtain prevents mixing of the ambient atmosphere with the sterile flow over the bed and sweeps away, downwards and outwards, any contaminant particles approaching the bed. Heaters are placed at the dual pre-filters to keep the air temperature around the patient at an appropriate level (usually 32 degrees of centigrade).

To test the efficiency of the machine in decontaminating the ward room, a bacteriological study was carried out after contaminating the room with a test microbe.

Methods

With the plant running continuously, the ward room was contaminated with a known quantity of Sarcina lutea (10^8). The microbes were dispersed in the room with an atomizer 2 meters over the floor (Fig. 2). Blood agar plates were placed on the bed, and on a table in the ward room. The distance from atomizer to both groups of plates was the same, and two persons uncovered the plates simultaneously. The air in the room was contaminated four times at fifteen minutes intervals, and samples for determination of bacterial counts were taken 1 and 5 minutes after every contamination, as well as 2 hours and 24 hours after the last contamination. The samples were taken when the bed was empty, and with a volunteer patient during rest and excercise, and during a mock nursing procedure. After incubation at 37 degrees of centigrade for 24 hours, the colonies on each plate were counted with an ordinary colony counter.

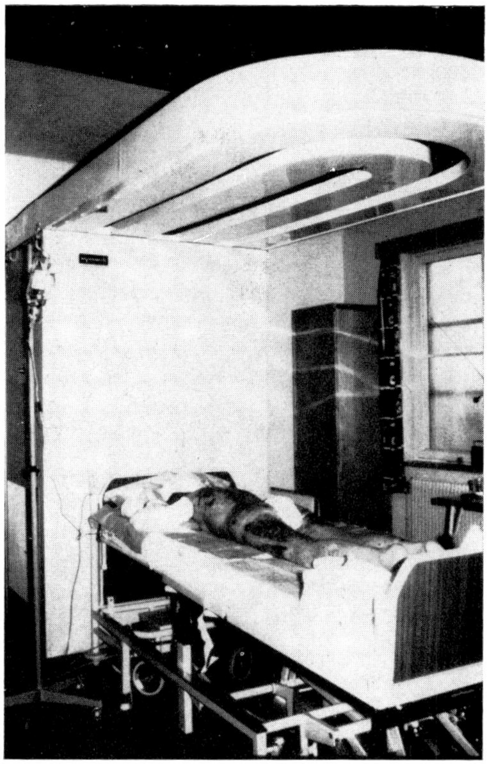

Fig. 1. Exposure treatment of patient in the STERAIR.

Results

The number of colonies on 3 plates in each trial was very close to each other, and the mean of 3 counts is considered representative (Fig. 3). In samples taken 1 minute after contamination the bacterial count behind the air curtain varied between 309 and 456, while the count on the outside varied between 1342 and 2113. Confluent growth was found on all plates exposed for 5 minutes. Fifteen minutes after the last contamination the bacterial count behind the air curtain was 82, and on the outside it was 134. Two hours after contamination the count behind the air curtain was reduced to zero, and on the outside to 3. No growth of the test microbe was found in any sample taken 24 hours after contamination.

Discussion

Despite heavy contamination of the ward room with the test microbe, there was a great difference between the bacterial count inside and outside the curtain, the ratio being about 1 : 4. The fact that the test microbe hardly could be found 2 hours after the last

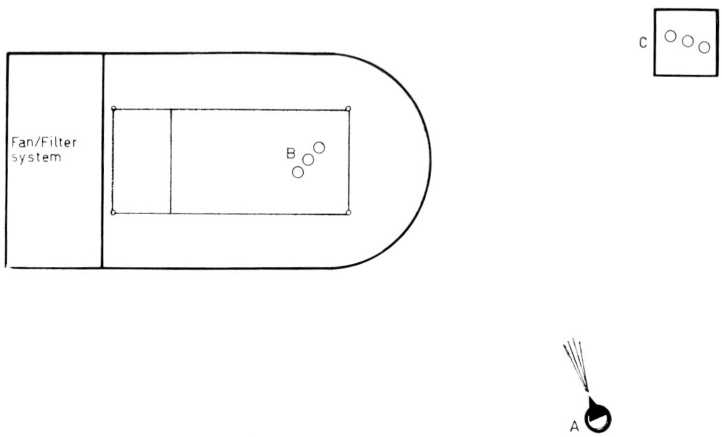

Fig. 2. Arrangement of experimental set-up.
(A — atomizer, B — blood agar plates on the bed. C — blood agar plates on table.)

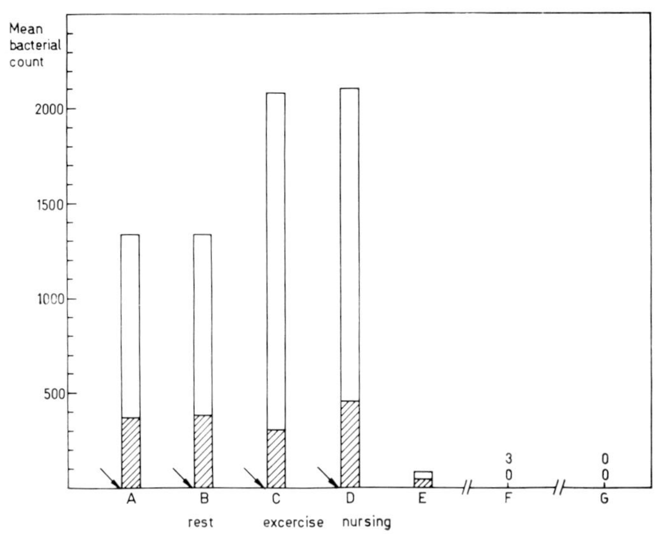

Fig. 3. Arrows indicate contamination with Sarcina lutea (10^8 microbes at 15 minutes intervals). (A, B, C, D — bacterial counts 1 minute after contamination. E — bacterial count 15 minutes after the last contamination. F and G — bacterial counts 2 respective 24 hours after contamination (see text). Hatched columns = bacterial counts behind the air curtain. White columns = bacterial counts in the ward room).

contamination is also noteworthy. Whether the volunteer was at rest, or was moving vigorously, seems to be of minor importance. A lower bacterial count from the samples behind the air curtain during excercise may be a mere coincidence, but it is most likely that some microbes escape through the air curtain at the floor, to be dispersed into the

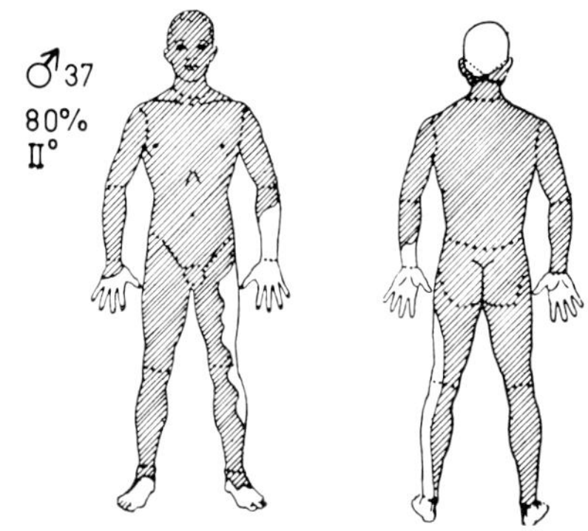

Fig. 4. Case 1. Man, age 37, with 80 per cent partial skin loss caused by scalding. Staph. aur. isolated from the burns on admission. Following exposure treatment in STERAIR for 16 days, cultures were negative. Successful grafting of two minor areas, and discharged 30 days postburn.

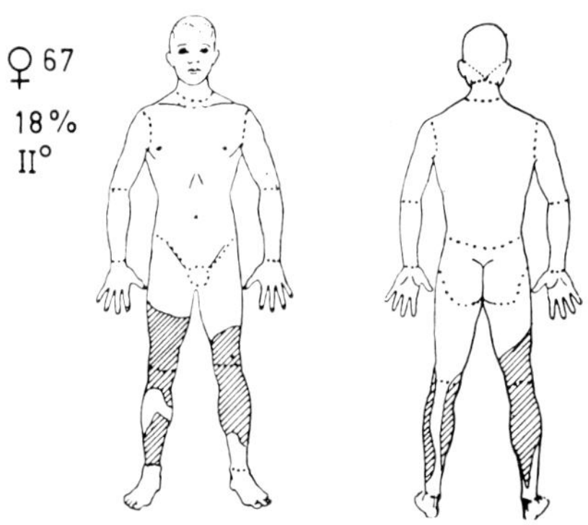

Fig. 5. Case 2. Woman, age 67, with 18 per cent partial skin loss caused by scalding of both lower extremities. Staph. aur. and E. coli isolated from the burns on admission. Exposure treatment in STERAIR for 13 days. The same strain of Staph. aur. demonstrable until spontaneous healing took place 16 days postburn. Discharged after 21 days in hospital.

ward room. This is in keeping with the comparatively high count in the room immediately after excercise. It is of course inevitable that the air curtain is broken several times during nursing procedures, a fact which possibly explains the higher count inside the air curtain as long as such activities are going on. There was, however, no striking increase of the count in the ward room during nursing procedures.

Our experience with the modified STERAIR is so far limited, since we have treated only 11 patients according to the principles just described. Nevertheless, we should like to report on two cases which might have offered great therapeutic problems if the treatment had been carried out according to our previous standard routine.

The bacteriological findings in our study are ample proof of the efficiency of the STER-AIR in decontaminating the air, especially in the ward room, but also around the patient. This decontaminating power, together with the exposure of the patient to a warm air flow, seems to be a good help in the treatment of severe burns.

O. M. U., Plastikkirurgi,
Tuengen Allé 7,
Vinderen,
Oslo 3, Norway

DETECTION OF ENDOTOXIN IN HUMAN PLASMA USING LIMULUS TEST

Z. KONÍČKOVÁ, J. SEDLÁK, V. MATĚJÍČEK, J. MORÁVEK and R. VRABEC

Burns Unit, Charles University, Prague, Laboratory of Plastic Surgery, Academy of Sciences, Centre of Clinical Pharmacology, Institute of Clinical and Experimental Medicine, Prague, Czechoslcvakia

The role of endotoxin in the development of manifest septicaemia has yet not been defined, because, until the recent past, no effective method for the detection of endotoxemia existed. This situation changed after Levin's Limulus test was introduced.

The Limulus test is a new method based on the gelation of Limulus amoebocytes lysate in the presence of minute amounts of endotoxin (2, 3). This effect probably represents a primitive defense of the organism against infection; the detailed mechanism of this process is as yet unknown. The reaction is specific for endotoxin, it cannot be triggered by other bacterial toxins.

The authors tested the sensitivity of the method in non-protein media and some modifications of this method for protein media, i.e. for human plasma. Finally, endotoxin detection was carried out on a series of plasma samples from patients with extensive burns.

In all experiments, the lysate from Marine Biological Laboratories, Woods Hole, and Difco endotoxin were used. Apyrogenic water, a pH 7.2 buffer and plasma ultrafiltrate served as non-protein media. Protein medium, human plasma, was obtained from heparinized blood.

The inhibitory effect of plasma proteins on the gelation was eliminated by chloroform extraction, by 1 : 40 plasma dilution or by a pH shift following Rheinhold and Fine (4).

In non-protein media, firm gelation occured at 10^{-10} g/ml endotoxin concentration. An incomplete gelation was observed at a concentration as low as 5.10^{-11} g/ml. At 10^{-11} g/ml concentration, the reaction could not be positively qualified.

In a protein medium, in human plasma, the inhibitory effect of plasma proteins on gelation could not be totally eliminated by the methods described above. The sensitivity of the method in plasma was about one hundred times lower than in non-protein media.

The results obtained with the use of the three modifications of the method for plasma did not markedly differ. With chloroform extraction and with plasma dilution endotoxin could be detected at 10^{-8} g/ml, with pH shift the reaction was positive at 5.10^{-9} g/ml endotoxin concentration (Table 1).

Better results could be obtained if the pH shift was followed by 1 : 10 plasma dilution. This experience was obtained when testing plasma samples from patients with extensive burns, where the inhibitory influence of plasma proteins seems to be expecially strong

TABLE 1

Detection of endotoxin using Limulus test

Endotoxin g/ml	Non-protein media		Human plasma				
	buffer pH 7.2	plasma ultrafiltr.	native	dilution 1 : 40	chlorof. extract.	phH shift	pH shift 1 : 10 dilut.
10^{-5}	+	+		+	+	+	+
10^{-6}	+	+		+	+	+	+
10^{-7}	+	+		+	+	+	+
10^{-8}	+	+		+	+	+	+
5.10^{-9}	+	+				+	+
10^{-9}	+	+					
10^{-10}	+	+		negative			
5.10^{-11}	+	+					

(probaly due to changes in protein patterns observed in burned patients) and could not be eliminated by a pH shift only.

In the first four cases out of eleven only the pH shift was used. The results were negative, though in two cases clinical manifestations pointed to endotoxic shock. In seven cases tested later, the pH shift was followed by 1 : 10 plasma dilution and the reaction was positive in all 5 suspect cases.

Summarizing their results, the authors reached the conclusion that the Limulus test is the first method that can be successfully used for endotoxin detection in burned patients. The impact of this method in pathophysiological studies of shock and septicaemia is self-evident; the diagnostic and prognostic importance of this method will have to be defined in the future.

References

1. Levin, J., Poore, T. E., Young, N. S., Margolis, S., Zauber, N. P., Townes, A. S., Bell, W. R. (1972): Gram-negative sepsis: detection of endotoxemia with the Limulus test. Ann. intern. Med. 76 : 1.
2. Levin, J., Poore, T. E., Zauber, N. P., Oser, R. S. (1970): Detection of endotoxin in the blood of patients with sepsis due to gram-negative bacteria. New Engl. J. Med. 283 : 1313.
3. Levin, J., Tomasulo, P. A., Oser, R. S. (1970): Detection of endotoxin in human blood and demonstration of an inhibitor. J. Lab. clin. Med. 75 : 903.
4. Reinhold, R. B., Fine, J. (1971): A technique for quantitative measurement of endotoxin in human plasma. Proc. Soc. exp. Biol. (N.Y.) 137 : 334.

Z. K., Legerova 63,
120 00 Praha 2, Czechoslovakia

COMPLICATIONS OF THE BURN ILLNESS

THE SICK CELL SYNDROME IN BURNS

D. M. JACKSON

Birmingham Accident Hospital, Great Britain

The Sick Cell Syndrome is a hypothesis rather than established fact, but it is a concept which is of considerable clinical value. It is a collection of biochemical and clinical changes which are attributed to impairment of some of the functions of the cell membrane. This disorder is due in turn to some general factor such as tissue anoxia. The syndrome is therefore not peculiar to burns but occurs also in thoracic injury and disease, circulatory insufficiency leading to tissue underperfusion, septicaemia and situations where there is a lack of calories or the ability to use them.

One of the functions of the cell membrane is to preserve the difference in concentration of sodium inside and outside the cell. The action of extruding sodium out of the cell entails metabolic energy, and has been likened to the action of 'a sodium pump'. This idea was first conceived by Dean in 1940 and has received much attention since (5). The sick cell syndrome is a clinical picture which might be expected from a failure of the sodium pump, but this has not yet been established due to the difficulty of measuring intracellular electrolytes.

A Typical Case

In a typical case, a patient with a 50 per cent burn who has got through the shock stage satisfactorily is progressing uneventfully for a week or more. He has received a liberal intake of water to cover extra losses through the burn and lungs (these are estimated by Davies at about 0.3 ml/sq.cm. of burn/day), and sufficient sodium to cover his normal requirements (120 mEq/day) plus the obligatory loss in the exudate (estimated by Davies at about 0.03 mEq/sq.cm. of burn/day when the burn is treated with silver nitrate or silver sulfadiazine creams). He has been receiving potassium at about the rate lost in the urine, as measured by 24 hour collections.

Then, one day, the biochemical investigations show a fall of serum sodium to 120—130 mEq/L; the Na/K ratio in the urine changes from 2/1 to less than 1/1, and next day, perhaps, sodium exretion in the urine drops to less than 10 mEq/L. The assumption is that sodium is passing into the general cells of the body with water, chloride and hydrogen ions, leading to an intracellular acidosis, and potassium is being lost from the cells and passed in the urine. When this picture begins, the patient has no complaints or physical signs; but two or three days later it will be noticed that he is confused and perhaps hyperventilating. If the patient is thin his ribs which are obvious initially become less so, because they are now covered with non-pitting, intracellular oedema. Untreated, this condition may progress steadily to a fatal outcome, with increasing confusion, hyperventilation and intracellular acidosis leading to failure of the heart, liver and kidneys.

When the clinician sees this low serum sodium with no sodium in the urine, he should resist the temptation to increase the sodium intake (provided, that is, the patient has been getting an average sodium intake, and has had extra supplements of sodium if he has been treated with silver nitrate compresses). Increased sodium intake in this condition fails to raise the sodium level in the serum or the urine; it only drives more sodium into the cells. Elderly people especially can be hastened to a fatal outcome by increasing salt intake to raise the serum sodium figure. What is needed is to get the sodium out of the cells again, and out of the body in the urine.

For several years now we have monitored the sodium in each 24-hour urine sample in all big burns, and we have recorded haemoglobin and serum electrolyte investigations once or twice weekly. This biochemical monitoring gives early warning of the development of the sick cell syndrome and an opportunity to prevent it.

The commonest cause of the disorder is hypovolaemia which, in our experience, tends to recur every week or two in the progress of a large burn. The low blood volume involves both the red cell mass and the plasma volume, so that haemoglobin and haematocrit estimations are nearly normal and give a poor guide to the blood volume. Direct measurement of the blood volume, using red cells tagged with radioactive chromium, often shows a loss of 20–30 per cent of the blood volume in the presence of a near normal haemoglobin.

Septicaemia is the other common cause of the syndrome, and in our experience the fall of urinary sodium to single figures has often been the first pointer to this complication.

Treatment

Prophylaxis. I have said that the biochemical changes are an early warning system, and since we have used them as such we have rarely seen the full clinical picture of the syndrome. The biochemical changes should arrest the clinician's attention and make him ask, "Is this patient suffering from hypovolaemia, septicaemia or some other stress, such as, anoxia, excessive cooling or under-nutrition. It is the patient not his biochemistry that needs treatment.

Therapy. Ideally, a firm diagnosis should precede treatment. If a blood volume estimation is not available, a transfusion of a quarter of the patient's blood volume is probably indicated to correct hypovolaemia which is the commonest cause.

Correction of the cause is always the first step: without this, other complications will snowball and the condition progress. Often this is sufficient alone, and in one or two days the fully developed clinical syndrome may disappear. But with very ill patients, and especially in the elderly, it may be worth giving further supportive treatment in the form of potassium, with glucose and insulin to drive it into the cells. This encourages release of the intracellular sodium and corrects intracellular acidosis (1, 3, 4).

Potassium, glucose and insulin (P.G.I.) is best given as a short intravenous infusion over 10–15 minutes of each hour from one bottle (Bottle A), and for the rest of each hour the same cannula can be used with a Y-junction for a bottle of 5 per cent dextrose in water or an intravenous feeding solution (Bottle B.). The P.G.I. solution is a 500 ml bottle of 25 per cent Glucose, to which is added 1000 units of Heparin, 10 mEq of potassium (as potassium chloride) and 28 units of soluble insulin; 100 ml of this is given hourly for one or two days. If there is any suggestion of a hypoglycaemic reaction from Bottle A, the infusion is switched at once to Bottle B — 'the safe bottle'. The aim is to keep the blood sugar at 140–160 per cent (measured by Dextristix), and a trace of sugar in the urine (measured by Clinistix). The first is done by the doctor at the end of each hour until the patient is stabilised, and then no further pricks are necessary: the second is continued hourly by the nurse for the period of the infusion. The patient may need slightly more or less insulin than advised initially, but once stabilised, the amount of insulin usually remains constant. As a check, one laboratory blood sugar estimation is advisable when sugar in the urine is a trace.

In conclusion, I would repeat that whether the present conception of the mechanism of the sick cell syndrome is eventually confirmed or not, the hypothesis of what may be happening is at present a valuable aid in the management of many large burns.

References

1. Allison, S. P., Hinton, P. and Chamberlain, M. J. (1968): Intravenous glucose-tolerance, insulin, and free-fattyacid levels in burned patients. Lancet 2 : 1113.
2. Davies, J. W. L. (1973): Personal communication.
3. Hinton, P., Allison, S. P., Farrow, S., Littlejohn, S. and Lloyd, J. (1972): Blood-volume changes and transfusion requirements of burned patients after the shock phase of injury. Lancet 1 : 913.
4. Hinton, P., Allison, S. P., Littlejohn, S., Lloyd, J. (1971): Insulin and glucose to Rudnee catabolic response to injury in burned patients. Lancet 1 : 767.
5. Thomas, R. C. (1972): Electrogenic sodium pump in nerve and muscle cells. Physiol. Rev. 52 : 563.

D. M. J., 29 Hamilton Avenue,
Harborene,
Birmingham 17, Great Britain

ACUTE FUNCTIONAL AND MORPHOLOGICAL ALTERATIONS AFTER SCALDING WITH SPECIAL REGARD TO THE LUNG: AN EXPERIMENTAL STUDY

H. WOLF, H. NEUHOF and D. HEY

Medical Clinics and Policlinics, Justus-Liebig University, Giessen, F.R.G.

Looking for a model which would reveal distinct pathologic pulmonary alterations within a short period of time we chanced on the model of acute scalding. In the following I will describe the hemodynamic and pulmonary alterations produced by scalding the caudal body-half of rabbits and the resulting changes in pulmonary histology.

23 rabbits weighing 2–3 kilograms each were anesthetized with Nembutal^{R}, relaxed with Imbretil^{R}, tracheotomized and isovolumetrically ventilated with normal air. Arterial blood pressure, pressure in the right ventricle and ventilation pressure were continuously measured by electromanometer and the values recorded. In addition oxygen uptake was continuously measured according to Neuhof's method. Cardiac output was determined by the thermo-dilution method in intervals of 2.5 to 15 minutes, and 0.5 milliliter arterial blood was taken to determine the following parameters: pH, carbon dioxide pressure, oxygen pressure, hemoglobin, hematocrit and oxygen saturation. Scalding was effected by pouring approximately 2 liters of 80°C hot water containing a detergent over the caudal body half of the animals for exactly 1 minute.

If scalding is too massive the animal dies of acute right heart failure within a maximum of 10 minutes. If the trauma is tolerated the following results are obtained:

Arterial blood pressure on the whole shows almost no changes (Fig. 1). There may be a slight rise, or — as in this case — a slight decrease. Pressure in the right ventricle distinctly rises within 3–5 minutes, and remains elevated for approximately 20 minutes. Ventilation pressure rapidly rises after a short incisure and then keeps rising continuously. This ventilation pressure is a direct reflection of pulmonary elasticity. If the pressure-volume curve is recorded by an xy-recorder (Fig. 2) a distinct rise in ventilation pressure is already seen after 2.5 minutes, and even more marked after 5 minutes. This curve is not remarkably influenced by the ventilation frequency of 45/min. The curve pattern remains the same also with extremely slow inspiration.

Cardiac output rapidly drops (Fig. 3) after a short increase and retains its decreasing tendency until death. Total peripheral resistance rises slowly and continuously as a reaction to reduced cardiac output. Oxygen uptake runs almost parallel to cardiac output. The decrease in oxygen uptake and cardiac output is mainly due to the massively increased resistance in the pulmonary circulation. A pressure increase in the right ventricle

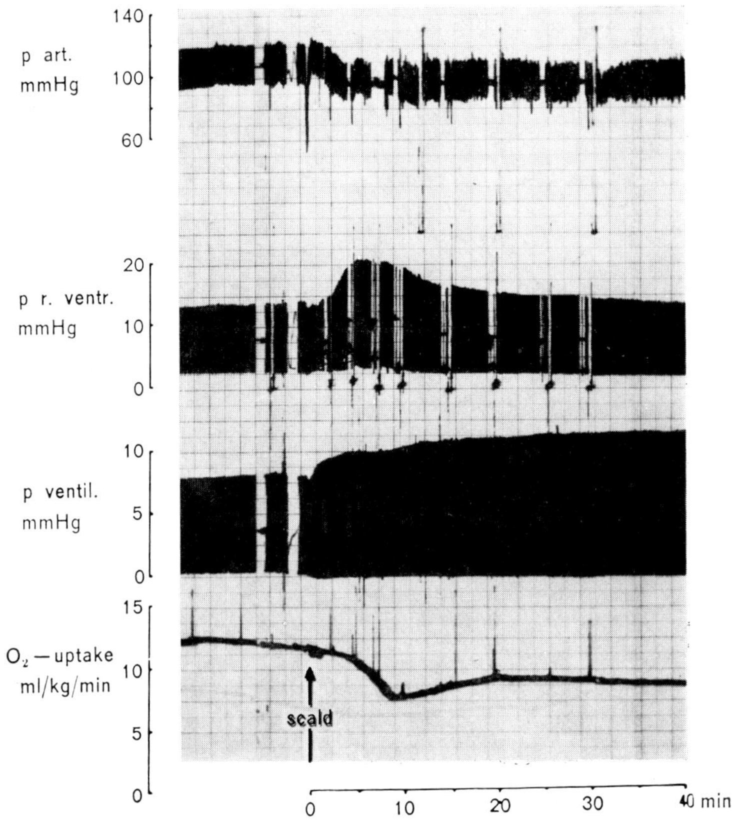

Fig. 1. Original registration strip showing arterial blood pressure (p art.), right ventricular pressure (p r. ventr.), ventilation pressure (p ventil.) and oxygen uptake before and after scald.

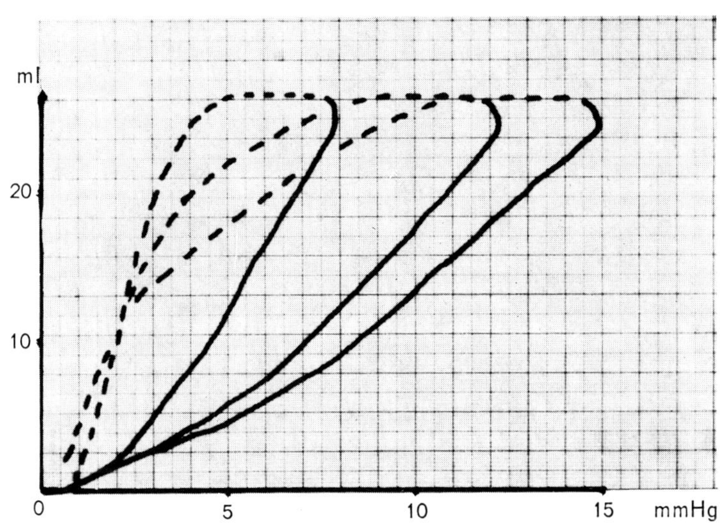

Fig. 2. Compliance before, 2.5, and 5 minutes after scald.

associated with reduced cardiac output without signs of left ventricular insufficiency indicates considerably increased resistance in the pulmonary vascular system. If the pressure in the left atrium is assumed to be constant, then the curve of pulmonary conductance (the reciprocal value of resistance) coincides with the curve of cardiac output. Accordingly, pulmonary resistance keeps increasing despite regressing pulmonary hypertension.

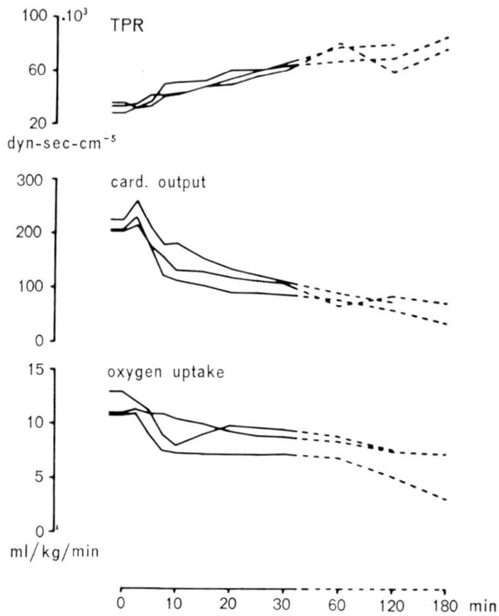

Fig. 3. Total peripheral resistance (TPR), cardiac output, and oxygen uptake after scald. (3 representative animals)

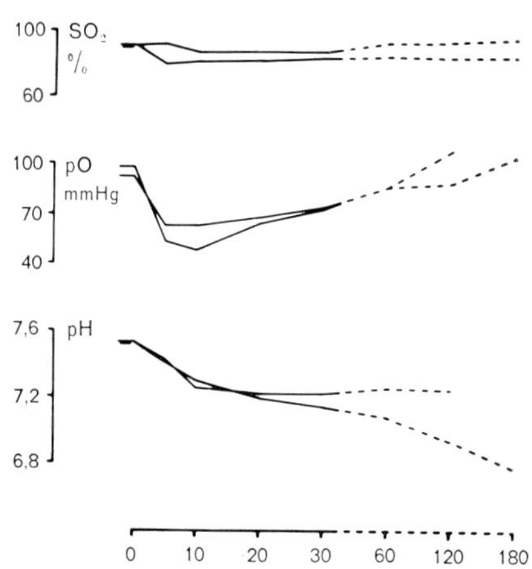

Fig. 4. Oxygen saturation (SO_2), oxygen pressure (pO_2), and pH in arterial blood after scald (2 representative animals).

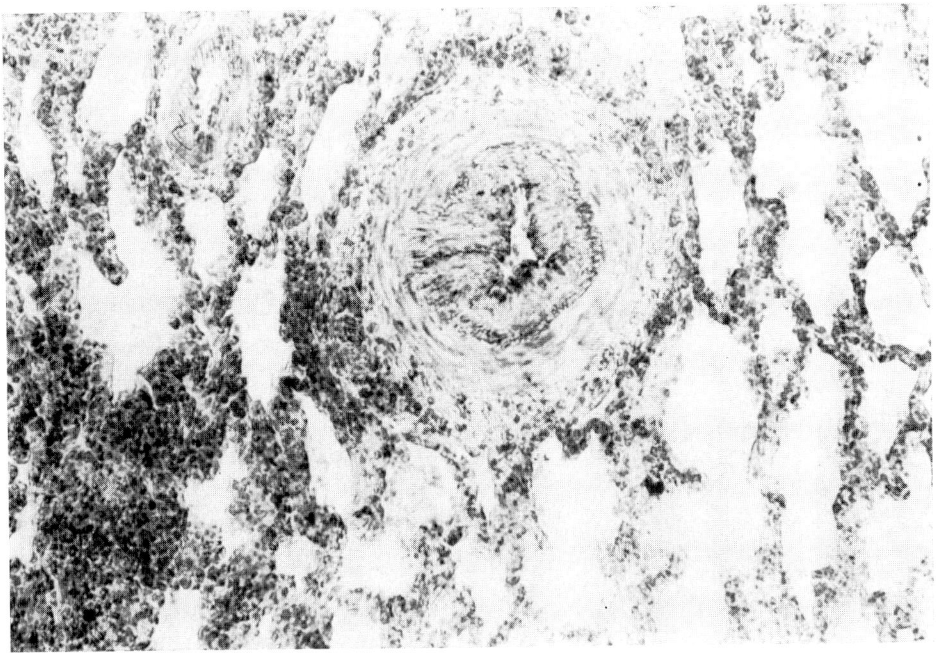

Fig. 5. Pneumonitis stage II: perivascular edema, interstitial edema, atelectasis.

After scalding arterial oxygen pressure decreases (Fig. 4) in a varying extent, but reaches its initial values again after 60 minutes at the latest. Arterial oxygen saturation, however, remains within the normal range (over 80 p.c.). With increasing acidosis this is in contradiction to the Bohr effect. Therefore changes in the configuration of the erythrocytes or changes in the hemoglobin molecule cannot be excluded in this transient decrease of arterial oxygen pressure. Braasch has demonstrated that changes in the membrane of the erythrocyte and an increase in volume are caused by severe burn. This is supported by the fact that we regularly observed hemolysis after scalding.

Independent of the survival time of the animals the histological specimen shows a shock lung pattern stage II (Fig. 5) (HEY) with perivascular and interstitial edema, atelectases and round cell infiltrates. Occasionally fibrinous fluid is found in small vessels and alveoli. These alterations are more pronounced near the hilus, whereas they may be almost absent in the periphery.

Using the same scalding model on the guinea pig, Romani already noted these histological changes in 1953 and ascribed them to the release of histamine. Clowes jr. produced identical histological changes in lung lobules perfused *in situ* with the blood of septic and hypovolemic dogs and held the following substances responsible: biogenic amines, ADP and prostaglandins, thrombin, the activated kinin system and other vasoactive peptides originating from the release of proteolytic lysosomal enzymes.

In principle, then histological lung pattern after acute scalding does not differ from that found in septic or traumatic shock, although the deterioration of pulmonary hemodynamics with its consequence on cardiac output could be best demonstrated in the model of acute scalding.

It may be assumed that in many forms of clinical shock increasing resistance in the pulmonary vascular system with the consecutive reduction of cardiac output below the minimum required for the oxygen supply of the organism is already of importance when the gas exchange function of the lung is still sufficient, although the development of the changes is not as pronounced and rapid as in the animal experiment. As already shown, massively increased resistance in the pulmonary vascular system accompanied by reduced cardiac output is not necessarily indicated by pulmonary hypertension.

References

1. Braasch, D. und Gössling, G. (1966): Erythrocytendeformierung und Quellung durch Plasmafaktoren nach schweren Verbrennungen. Pflügers Arch. ges. Physiol. 289 : 1.
2. Clowes, Ch. A., Jr. (1973): Die Wirkung posttraumatisch und bei Sepsis auftretender zirkulierender Peptide auf die Lunge. Med. Welt 24 (NF) : 1154.
3. Hey, D. (1971): Habilitationsschrift. Giessen
4. Neuhof, H. (1970): Habilitationsschrift. Giessen
5. Romani, J. D. (1953): Les lésions pulmonaires au cours des brûlures expérimentales chez le cobaye. C. r. Soc. Biol. (Paris) 147 : 262.

H. W., Med. Kliniken,
Klinikstr. 32b,
63 Giessen, F.R.G.

RESPIRATORY COMPLICATIONS IN THE EARLY POST BURN PERIOD

C. C. M. HOWIE

Bangour General Hospital, Broxburn, West Lothian, Great Britain

Respiratory complications arising early in the post-burn period present a problem in differential diagnosis. The temptation to attribute all of them to the effects of heat or smoke must be resisted. They may be due to cerebral disaster, to acute or chronic cardio-respiratory disease or to an excessive intake of alcohol or depressant drugs prior to injury. Iatrogenic factors such as overinfusion, over-sedation or poor general management may also be responsible. In many cases, there is more than one aetiological factor.

A seven year old boy was admitted three hours after he had sustained 76 per cent deep burns. He had already had two injections each of 10 mgs. morphia intravenously. He had severe airway obstruction from thermal damage and immediate tracheostomy was necessary. Three hours later, respirations became slow and irregular. The pCO_2 was 50 mmHg. Intravenous nalorphine produced immediate improvement.

A 63 year old man was admitted three hours after he sustained 17 p.c. superficial burns including the face. His respirations were shallow, he was disorientated, noisy and unco-operative. He was given 10 mgs. of Diazepam intravenously. There were carbon particles in his mouth but none in his trachea. He was put on assisted ventilation with 40 p.c. oxygen through an endotracheal tube. A further 10 mg of Diazepam was given. On this, his pH was 7.30, pO_2 146 mmHg, pCO_2 45 mmHg. Over the next few hours, he became unconscious. The respiratory rate fell to 6 per minute and respiration had to be controlled. He gradually took over his own respiration, became conscious and co-operative. At 32 hours post injury, his pCO_2 was 50 mm when breathing air spontaneously. At 56 hours the tube was removed and thereafter he maintained acceptable blood/gas tensions. It was only after he had been with us for 30 hours that we learned that he had been given a presumably sizeable quantity of brandy, Pethidine 50 mg intravenously, and 100 mg intramuscularly prior to his transfer to us. He may have inhaled some smoke but his respiratory problem was primarily due to the depressant drugs obtained from three separate sources in the first 6 hours.

A 46 year old lady weighing 49 kg with 12 p.c. deep burns involving the face was rescued unconscious from a smoke filled hall. Soon after her admission to hospital, her systolic blood pressure fell to 60 mm. Over about the next three hours, 1.5 litres of plasma and 800 ml of crystalloid were given intravenously. The systolic rose to 110 mm but following this, she developed signs of pulmonary oedema. She was given a diuretic' intubated and ventilated with 100 p.c. oxygen. On this, her pH was 7.15, pCO_2 68 mm. Hg, SaO_2 91 p.c. (= pO_2 81 mmHg), standard bicarbonate 16.5 M. equiv/L. As her respiratory function improved, the oxygen percentage was reduced. On the 4th day, she was extubated and breathing spontaneously and by the 9th day, she was off oxygen. She had no antibiotic and after the first day, no bronchodilator drugs (2). She was transferred to the Burn Unit three days later. She was disorientated, cyanosed and dyspnoeic with marked bronchospasm and copious secretions. On oxygen 3 litres by Edinburgh Mask (29–41 p.c.) the pH 7.480, pO_2 82 mmHg, pCO_2 41.3 mmHg. She was treated with antibiotics, physiotherapy, bronchodilators, humidity and oxygen. Three days later, breathing air, pO_2 62.5 and after a further four days, had risen to 72 mmHg. This patient probably suffered lung damage from smoke but her initial infusion therapy was excessive in relation to her weight and the size of her burn. The more so in that she had had a mitral valvotomy 14 years before and was on Digoxin for auricular fibrillation. Her chest X-ray constantly showed cardiac enlargement and pulmonary venous hypertension. She died from blockage of her mitral valve 6 weeks after her discharge from our unit.

A workman sustained deep burns of the face from an oxyacetylene blow lamp. He also had a small burn on the right thigh. There was blistering of the tip of the tongue and a few carbon particles were found on tracheal suction. At 24 hours on oxygen 3 litres, the pH was 7.36, pO_2 88 mmHg, pCO_2 46 mmHg. Over the next 48 hours, still on the same therapy, the pO_2 progressively fell to 68 mmHg. He was very ill with signs indicating collapse of the left lung with accumulation of secretions. X-rays from the previous three days showed progressive diminution of air entry on the left side. Contrary to our usual practice, a new junior had instructed that the burn of the thigh had to be kept uppermost at all times. For 4 days, his left lung had been dependent with secretions from his nasal burn draining into it. Immediate physiotherapy produced immediate improvement. With better general management, the lung re-expanded. 5 days later, he was off oxygen with a pO_2 of 88 mmHg.

A 41 year old man sustained 90 p.c. deep burns in an explosion in an electricity substation which filled with black smoke. His airway was clear and there were no adventitial sounds in the lungs. At 18 hours post burn, he was taken to theatre. Carbon particles were seen in the pharynx and endotracheal suction revealed gross carbon contamination. He was given preventive therapy. Apart from coughing up carbon-stained sputum for two days, he developed no signs relative to his respiratory tract.

A seaman was dragged unconscious from his smoke filled cabin and admitted with 10 p.c. superficial burns of face and arms. He was restless and had bronchospasm and rales over both lungs. The soft palate was blistered and he was coughing up carbon-stained sputum. His pH 7.44, pO_2 62 mmHg, pCO_2 35 mmHg, standard bicarbonate 24.5 m.equ/L. He was given high humidity and started on bronchodilator therapy and an antibiotic. Immediate physiotherapy produced such clinical improvement that oxygen was withheld and his blood gases repeated 6 hours later. The pO_2 was 58 mmHg and for the next 7 days he had to be given continuous oxygen 3 litres, by the Edinburgh Mask. Oxygen therapy was finally stopped on the 12th day when his pO_2 was 70 mmHg.

This old lady was more severely affected. Carbon impregnation could be seen in the 10 p.c. superficial burns of face and shoulders. There was no heat damage within the mouth. There were some course rales in the lungs. She was put on general preventive therapy and 3 litres of oxygen. 6 hours later, the pO_2 was 73 mmHg, pCO_2 42 mmHg. At 14 hours post injury, she developed pulmonary oedema and had to be put on assisted ventilation with 40 p.c. oxygen via an endotrachael tube. As two attempts to take her off I.P.P.V. (intermittent positive pressure ventilation) had resulted in recurrence of pulmonary oedema, a tracheostomy was done on the 6th day when her pO_2 off the ventilator was still only 52 mm. Her pO_2 started to rise on the 10th day and weaning from the ventilator was complete by the 18th day when her pO_2 was 65 mmHg. By the 20th day, the pO_2 was 76 mmHg. Her tracheostomy tube was removed on the 24th day.

These patients illustrate some of the respiratory complications which the clinician may encounter in the early post-burn period. Many of these are avoidable. Too high or too frequent dosage with narcotic drugs will inevitably cause respiratory depression. This may appear later and last longer that one expects. The risk of pulmonary oedema from over-infusion is very real. Every burned patient requires frequent changes of position and respiratory physiotherapy if pulmonary complications are to be avoided. This is even more necessary if the nose or mouth is involved in the burn and a close watch must be kept in the early period for the signs of airway obstruction. If smoke damage to the lung is suspected, blood gas analysis should be done repeatedly in the first 48 hours. Sedation should be minimal and over-infusion avoided. The inspired air should be humidified, physiotherapy started and a course of antibiotic and bronchodilator drugs given. These measures are adequate for some patients. In a more severely affected patient, oxygen therapy may be required. Intravenous bronchodilators and Cortisone in high dosage (1) may be necessary to relieve bronchospasm and prevent bronchial mucosal oedema. I.P.P.V. may have to be instituted to raise the oxygen tension or to control pulmonary oedema. Blood gases should be done on oxygen therapy to ensure that it is effective and that the patient is not being subjected to too high oxygen tension. The patient's progress should be assessed by blood gas analysis off oxygen therapy.

Blood gas tensions are essential in the differential diagnosis of respiratory complications. In alveolar damage from smoke, the pO_2 will be lowered. The pCO_2 is also lowered and the pH is high. If pulmonary oedema or stasis of secretions develops, there will be a rise in the pCO_2 and a further fall in the pO_2. In airway obstruction, there will be a progressive marked rise in the pCO_2, the pH will fall and later the pO_2. By then a clinical diagnosis should have been made. In respiratory depression from drugs, the pCO_2 will also be raised. The extent of the rise and whether the pO_2 is affected depends on the severity of the depression. In the inital shock phase of an extensive burn, there is an increase in physiological dead space (2). The pO_2 and the pCO_2 both fall but there is a metabolic acidosis and a low pH. In the weeks subsequent to injury, all extensively burned patients have a low pCO_2 and a high pH but usually no serious hypoxia (4). In the presence of multiple aetiological factors, the pCO_2 can be a useful guide to the cause of hypoxia.

References

1. Di Vincenti, F. C. et al. (1971): Inhalation injuries. J. Trauma 11 : 109.
2. Freeman, J. and Nunn, J. (1963): Ventilation-perfusion relationships after haemorrhage. Clin. Sci. 24 : 135.
3. Lloyd, E. L. and MacRae, W. R. (1971): Respiratory tract damage in burns. Brit. J. Anaesth. 43 : 365.
4. Pruitt, B. A., Jr. et al. (1970): Pulmonary complications in burn patients. J. thor. cardiovasc. Surg. 59 : 7.

C. C. M. H., Bangour General Hosp., Broxburn, West Lothian, Great Britain

RENAL DISEASE IN SEVERE BURNS

J. PETRÁSEK, R. KÖNIGOVÁ and J. ŠTEFAN

Institute of Clinical Physiology, Charles University, Prague
Burns Center, University Hospital, Prague
Institute of Forensic Medicine, Charles University, Prague, Czechoslovakia

An adequate intravenous fluid therapy of the burn shock considerably lowered the number of renal insufficiencies. The available data about renal involvement as a complicating factor in severe burn injury are sparse or not available. Our follow-up study therefore sought to answer the following problems:

1. Does there still develop any serious disorder of the kidney function under improved conditions of adequate fluid intake?
2. If we find a frequent incidence of renal complications we want to identify:
   a) what kind of disorder is the most frequent;
   b) the possible onset of renal disturbance in the altering course of the burn disease;
   c) the pathogenetic mechanisms involved, and the possibility of prevention.

The severely burned patients admitted to our intensive care ward in the Prague Burns Center over the past few years were treated in line with the same general principles of reanimation and general therapy. We studied 255 patients hospitalized from 1971 to 1973 (Table 1).

As an indication of a functional renal disturbance we used the increasing level of serum

TABLE 1

Severe burns treated in 1971–73

Total number of patients with 2nd–3rd degree burns over 20 per cent of the body surface	255
Survived	190
Died	65

TABLE 2

Total numbers of kidney involvement

Total number of severely burned patients with renal complications	76
Survived	50
Died	26

TABLE 3

Renal pathology in 26 burn fatalities

Histological findings	Number of patients
Acute tubular necrosis	16
Acute non-suppurative inflammations	
a) acute diffuse glomerulonephritis	1
b) acute focal glomerulonephritis	3
c) subacute glomerulonephritis	2
Acute suppurative inflammations	
a) abscesses in the cortex	2
b) abscesses in the medulla	2
Total	26

creatinin and blood urea. At the same time we followed the onset of proteinuria, the urine sediment, the bacteriology of the urine. Of the 76 afflicted, 50 patients with renal damage recuperated and 26 died (Table 2).

The character of the injury was similar in both groups, i.e. involvement of 20–90 p.c. of the body surface of the deep 2nd, 3rd and 4th degrees. In the fatalities, the pathologist informed us about the histological findings of the kidney. The total number of patients who died after the burn injury, in which the autopsy established pathological kidney changes, was 26. We classified this group according to prevalent morphological changes (Table 3).

Acute tubular necrosis was the most frequent finding, i.e. in 16 burned patients, and acute non-suppurative inflammation was detected in 6 patients with renal complications. Acute suppurative inflammations were observed in 4 patients, 2 of whom had abscesses in the cortex and in 2 the medulla was damaged — without any previous history of urological disorder.

In all 16 patients with tubular necrosis (Table 4) we found, from the very start marked proteinuria, erythrocytes in urine sediment and haemoglobinuria or myoglobinuria in patients No. 3, 4, 9, 10, 11.

In 6 patients with non-suppurative kidney inflammations (Table 5), proteinuria was positive after a certain time-period in each of them. Patient No. 17, 19, 20 showed erythrocytes in the urine sediment and No. 21 and 22 granular casts. There was constant bacteriological finding of Staphylococcus pyogenes aureus on the burned area.

Table 6 reviews 4 patients with suppurative inflammations. Abscesses in the cortex were found in patients No. 23 and 24, abscesses in the medulla in patients No. 25 and 26. The common finding was Staphylococcus pyogenes aureus in combination with Pseudomonas aeruginosa.

Discussion

The nephrologically oriented analysis of the severe burns in our care shows that the kidney complications occur in various forms in severe burns. While definite renal insufficiency was found in only 3 patients, i.e. 1.17 p.c. of all those treated, we must still expect that infusion and antishock therapy can be delayed by many causes. One of the main causes of the prolonged shock period or of its irreversible course is a late onset of the entire shock treatment. On the other side, histological findings in kidney with serious changes amounting to tubular necrosis do not exclude the possibility of satisfactory renal

TABLE 4

Acute tubular necrosis

Patient's Number	Age	Percentage of the burned surface	No. of days of treatment	Clinical course	Antibiotics	N-urea mg/100 ml of plasma	Creatinine mg/100 ml of plasma
1	32	54	14	sepsis, endotoxic shock	gentamycin polymyxin	35	2.1
2	37	50	14	resp. tract involvement septicemia	gentamycin	37	2.0
3	73	30	14	carbonisation of the limbs anuria		117	8.5
4	57	80	2	resp. tract involvement haematemesis		70	
5	41	65	2	resp. tract involvement, physical exertion after injury	kanamycin tetracyclin	65	
6	32	54	12	prolonged shock sepsis	pyopen	46	2.5
7	51	90	4	chemical burn	chfn	112	6.0
8	70	32	9	electrical burn haematemesis melaena		33	1.3
9	48	95	6	transport without antishock therapy	gentamycin	66	1.9
10	56	60	4	transport without antishock therapy		140	9.0
11	65	15 (4th degree)	9	electric burn sepsis	gentamycin oxacillin	35	1.8
12	51	65	8	obesity, sepsis	oxacillin	58	1.8
13	17	32	4	prolonged shock Pickwick's syndrome		19,5	1.1
14	23	30	15	transport without antishock therapy, sepsis	gentamycin septrin	79	2.2
15	3	60	7	prolonged shock, haematemesis, sepsis	gentamycin oxacillin	45	0,95
16	49	55	20	prolonged shock sepsis	gentamycin oxacillin	127	1.8

function. Acute tubular necrosis must be considered above all in cases when, right after the injury, proteinuria and erythrocytes occur, and the level of creatinin and urea in the blood plasma gradually rises. Haemoglobinuria and myoglobinuria are found

TABLE 5

Non-suppurative inflammations of the kidney

Patient's No.	Age	Percentage of the burned surface	No. of days of treatment	Comments on the clinical course	Bacteriology	N-urea mg/100 ml	Creatinine mg/100 ml
17	45	40	7	St. p. carditis rheumatica; hyperthermia 2nd day	Staph. pyog. aur. Pseudomonas	40	2.0
18	18	80	10	hyperthermia 5th day	Staphyl. pyog. aur. Pseudomonas	55	1.9
19	56	60	14	hyperthermia 3rd day	Staphyl. pyog. aureus	48	2.1
20	59	27	18	resp. tract involvement, tracheotomy, hyperthermia 5th day	Staphyl. pyog. aureus Pseudomonas	84 85	4.5
21	72	21	45	alcohol addict, sepsis	Staphyl. pyog. aureus	65	3.5
22	17	55	46	sepsis	Pseudomonas Achromobacter Staphyl. pyog. aureus	69	3.0

TABLE 6

Suppurative inflammations of the kidney

Patient's Number	Age	Percentage of burned surface	No. of days of treatment	Comments on the clinical course	Bacteriology	Proteinuria	N-urea	Creatinine
23	47	54	18	resp. tract involvement tracheotomy hyperthermia 2nd day	Staphyl. pyog. aureus Pseudomonas	2nd day starting	46	1.4
24	23	50	17	electrical burn, hyperthermia 5th day, sepsis	Staphyl. pyog. aureus Pseudomonas	5th day starting	38	1.5
25	23	80	42	hyperthermia 2nd day, sepsis	Staph. pyog. aur. Pseudomonas	from the beginning	97	2.6
26	26	70	14	hyperthermia 3rd day, sepsis	Staphylococcus pyog. aur. Pseudomonas	7th day starting	75	1.9

in deep burns extending to the muscle layer. This is a deteriorating effect to the kidney involvement.

Another unfavourable factor in the course of the shock and the state of the kidney is protracted unsuitable transport of the injured patient, or physical exertion immediately after the injury.

In patients in the higher age group, increased sensitivity of the kidney during the shock period is ascribed to diminished vascular reactivity. In our group patients No. 3, 8, 11, 21 suffered from minor injury than the rest, but their kidneys were seriously damaged.

Increasing overall infection is commonly inherent to severe burns. It is necessary to apply antibiotics and vary them often because of the altered sensitivity of the microbes. Frequently, we cannot avoid the use of antibiotics with side-effect nephrotoxicity. After certain antibiotics an increasing number of acute renal damage is reported.

Circulatory derangement in the kidney can be followed, shortly after the injury, by inflammations. Of the non-suppurative inflammations, we met both forms of acute glomerulonephritis: the diffuse form in one case and the focal form three times. Bioptic examination performed by other authors shows the existence of continuous transitions from the focal form to the diffuse. Both are considered to be caused by immunological changes. One interesting finding was that of Staphylococcus pyogenes aureus in the throat right after the injury in cases of non-suppurative glomerulonephritis.

Embolic kidney inflammations occur in septicemia when the kidney is the most often involved organ. The kidney receives the highest proportion (of all organs in the body) of the cardiac output. While the kidney accounts for only 0.4 per cent of the body weight, it receives one quarter of the cardiac output.

Suppurative inflammations occurred in our patients with mixed Staphylococcus pyogenes aureus and Pseudomonas aeruginosa infections.

In the current work reviewed here we found that renal complications continue to exist as a frequent deteriorating disorder in severe burns despite meticulous efforts to improve the general care.

References

1. Artz, C. P., Fitts, T. C. (1962): Replacement therapy in shock. J. Trauma 2 : 358.
2. Holmes, J. H. (1963): Acute tubular necrosis and its management. Surg. Clin. N. Amer. 34 : 525.
3. Wilson, C. (1967): The natural history of nephritis. In: Renal Disease. Oxford, Blackwell Scient. Publ.
4. Research in Burns (1966). Transactions of the Second International Congress on Research in Burns, Edinburgh, Livingstone.
5. Research in Burns (1971). Transactions of the Third Internationa Congress on Research in Burns, Prague 1970. Huber, Bern.

J. P., Inst. of Clinical, Physiology,
Ke Karlovu 4,
120 00 Praha 2, Czechoslovakia

IMMUNOREACTIVE INSULIN, SOMATOTROPIN, RENIN, ANGIOTENSIN II, ACTH AND LH LEVELS IN SEVERELY BURNED PATIENTS

R. DOLEČEK, M. ZÁVADA, M. ADÁMKOVÁ and K. LEIKEP

Regional Hospital, Burns Unit, Department of Medicine, Department of Nuclear Medicine, Ostrava, Czechoslovakia

All major burns are accompanied by a more or less pronounced endocrine and metabolic response of the burned organism. The high antidiuretic hormone (ADH) serum levels, very increased catecholamine and corticoid excretion in urine in severely burned patients have been repeatedly described (for review see 1.5). In recent years a few papers have appeared dealing with the plasma immunoreactive insulin (IRI), somatotropin (STH) and renin (REN) levels after major burns (1, 3, 4, 6, 7, 8), the first report about ACTH levels is just being published (9).

In this communication the authors present some of their results with plasma IRI, STH, REN, angiotensin II (ANGIO II), ACTH and LH estimation in burned patients.

Methods

For all the above estimations, the radioimmunoassay kits from RCC, Amersham, England (IRI, ACTH) and Serono (LH) and Sorin (REN, ANGIO II, STH), Italy, have been used.

Blood samples were collected in the morning hours (07:00–08:00) into chilled tubes and the plasma samples were kept at −20 degrees of centigrade until processed. As functional tests for IRI release, the standard oral glucose tolerance tests (OGTT) were used, while the STH release was stimulated with intravenous crystalline insulin (0.1 unit per 1 kg of body weight). To stimulate the REN and ANGIO II release, the patients were examined twice: after an overnight bedrest, and after 20 min. walking (if capable to walk).

Altogether 45 burned patients were examined, with a mean *burn index* (see 2) of 32.8.

Results and Discussion

If compared with the normal mean (17.7 ± 9.3 microU/ml), the mean IRI fasting levels of the burned patients (27 were examined) were increased for 7 postburn weeks. Their mean values ± S.D. were: 26.6 ± 14.8 (I-15); 36,5 ± 30,9 (II-12); 27,2 ± 26,4 (III-13); 42.2 ± 50.9 (IV-10); 40.3 ± 39.1 (V-10); 38.4 ± 27.9 (VI + VII-11);

TABLE 1

IRI levels (microU/ml) and blood glucose levels (mg/100 ml) in burned patients during glucose tolerance tests

Time in min. after the oral glucose load (g/kg)	I Normal controls (n = 10)	II All burned patients (n = 22)	III Patients with abnormal IRI and glucose response	Significance of differences between I and II, I and III
		immunoreactive insulin		
			(n = 10)	
0 min.	13.6 ± 3.8	17.0 ± 14.6	19.2 ± 21.5	n.s.
30 min.	36.4 ± 21.6	68.0 ± 55.5	108.6 ± 57.5	I and III ($p < 0.002$)
60 min.	44.8 ± 26.6	116.1 ± 170.8	212.4 ± 217.9	I and III ($p < 0.05$)
120 min.	27.3 ± 19.6	49.9 ± 71.6	103.2 ± 86.2	I and III ($p < 0.05$)
		blood glucose levels		
			(n = 7)	
0 min.	85.9 ± 12.3	76.2 ± 19.2	79.3 ± 27.1	n.s.
20 min.	129.7 ± 22.7	119.1 ± 33.6	145.9 ± 35.7	n.s.
60 min.	130.2 ± 34.7	129.4 ± 34.7	156.3 ± 27.3	n.s.
120 min.	86.9 ± 13.5	95.1 ± 27.6	126.1 ± 20.1	I and III ($p < 0.001$)

20.9 ± 9.3 (VIII + IX-9); 11.2 ± 6.4 microU/ml (X and more — 6). The values in parentheses indicate the postburn weeks and the number of patients examined. The mean blood glucose values were normal, except for the increased first week value and the decreased value of patients 10 weeks postburn and more. The IRI levels from the weeks I, II, V, VI + VII were significantly higher than the mean IRI fasting levels in normal controls (p less than 0.05 to p less than 0.01).

The decreased glucose tolerance and the increased insulin resistance are illustrated in Table 1. Most patients with a decreased glucose tolerance were from the first postburn weeks, while the increased IRI response during OGTT was not limited to those first postburn weeks.

The mean STH fasting levels after burns were somewhat increased, mainly in the second postburn month. But the STH plasma levels during the first two postburn weeks did not increase after a standard insulin load. Their means ± S.D. at 0 — 30 — 60 min. were: 1.9 ± 1.0 — 1.9 ± 0.85 — 3.3 ± 0.99 ng/ml. The blood glucose levels at the same time were: 91.6 ± 22.4 — 60.1 ± 35.5 — 59.6 ± 18.3 mg/100 ml. In the later postburn weeks, the STH response increased markedly, it was higher than in the normal controls: 4.2 ± ± 2.3 — 15.4 ± 11.5 — 10.2 ± 5.2 ng/ml, with their respective blood glucose levels: 80.8 ± 17.3 — 38.4 ± 12.3 — 56.6 ± 24.5 mg/100 ml. The "non-reactor" group includes 7 burned patients, while the other group includes 10 patients. In the normal control group (males) (n = 10) the STH levels were: 2.1 ± 0.9 — 3.7 ± 2.7 — 10.1 ± 3.3 ng/ml, with the blood glucose levels: 76.3 ± 23.5 — 32.9 ± 16.7 — 52.3 ± 25.0 mg/100 ml. The STH response in females is higher. It is interesting to note that in the same patient

TABLE 2

Plasma REN (ng/ml/hr) and ANGIO II (pg/ml) levels in 8 burned patients

Name, age, sex, burn index	Weeks after Burns I	II	III	IV	V + VI		REN ANGIO II
D.Z., 22, m	22.3	9.6	37.0	14.5	Died		
63 points	314	530	505	480			
N.A., 32, f	13.0	2.2	1.1	6.6	5.7	Died	
53 points	340	—	—	—	—		
		4.3					
M.M., 38, m	19.6	—	3.8	—	3.0		
52 points	270	—	235	—	125		
L.A., 42, f	—	—	1.9/7.0*				
37 points			470/420				
B.O., 49, f	—	—	—	—	5.8 /8,8*		
35 points					650/605		
Ř.M., 22, m	6.3	8.1	4.7	1.2			
33 points	415	660	290	355			
S.B., 32, m	—	—	—	2.7/4.7*			
24 points				400/370			
Z.L., 13, m	2.1	2.1					
18 points	235	450					
		1.1					
		340					

* recumbent/upright (20 min. walking)
Burn Index: each per cent of third degree burn represents 1 point, each per cent of second degree burn 1/2 point

Normal results from unburned controls (n = 10), recumbent/upright (± SD).
REN 1.5 ± 0.8/1.9 ± 1.1 ng/ml/hr; ANGIO II 153.2 ± 55.5/168.0 ± 52,1 pg/ml.
For more details and more results see (8).

TABLE 3

Plasma ACTH (pg/ml) and LH (mU/ml) levels in two burned patients

Name, age, sex burn index	Weeks after burns I		II		III	IV	V	The hormone studied
N.A., 32, f	430		170*	240**	180	—		ACTH
53 points			1200	580				
	26		7.0	7.0	6.7			LH
S.L., 32, m	220*	110**	40		10	70	230***	ACTH
28 points	350	20						
	22		10		12	13	22	LH

* before / after 3hr physiologic saline infusion
** before / after 3hr physiologic saline infusion + neuroplegic M2 mixture
*** septic fevers

the STH response changes significantly in the postburn weeks, when the same insulin dose is applied. E.g. *M.M., male, 38 yr, burn index 52.* STH response: 1.2 — 1.4 — 4.6 (I); — 1.8 — 7.5 — 12.6 (III); — 3.9 — 19.0 — 18,5 ng/ml (V), with the respective blood glucose levels: 118 — 100 — 79; 98 — 42 — 106; 106 — 44 — 64 mg/100 ml. The postburn weeks are in parentheses. *H.M., female, 48 yr, burn index 35.* STH response: 1.6 — 1.6 — 2.9 (II), 1.4 — 10.0 — 6.5 (XIII) ng/ml, with the blood glucose levels: 87 — 28 — 28 mg/100 ml and 68 — 28 — 36 mg/100 ml.

The fasting REN and ANGIO II plasma levels after major burns were always increased, and these high levels persisted in severely burned patients for more weeks (see Table 2). The increase was sometimes as high as twenty times the normal mean for plasma REN. The highest plasma REN level found was 37 ng/ml/hr, while the highest ANGIO II level was 660 pg/ml. The response of the renin-angiotensin system to the upright position in burned patients who just started to walk again was rather exaggerated. It could be compared with the response of adrenalectomized patients, e.g. 1.9/7.0/ng/ml/hr (recumbent/upright). The magnitude of the REN increase is not always parallel to the increase of ANGIO II levels.

The high plasma ACTH levels after major burns can persist for more postburn weeks (see Table 3). They can even reach the ACTH levels in patients with the central form of the Cushing's syndrome (e.g. 1200 pg/ml, as compared with the normal 10–80 pg/ml). In both patients included in Table 3, the high rise of ACTH plasma levels between 06:00 and 09:00 a.m. was more or less blocked when the neuroplegic M2 mixture was administered instead of the physiologic saline. The neuroplegic M2 mixture includes Sandosten-Calcium[R] (an antihistaminic) + Hydergin[R] (a partial alpha receptor blocking agent) + Panthesin[R] (similar to procaine).

The first results of LH estimation in plasma of severely burned patients during the first few postburn weeks, did not show any decrease. On the contrary, the LH plasma levels seemed to be increased in the first postburn week as if the peripheric endocrine gland had been damaged. Values as high as 26 mU/ml were found.

The above results can be used both clinically and to understand better the pathophysiology of the burn disease. We advocate the use of crystalline insulin in the first postburn days when glucose is administered (6.7) intravenously (e.g. 1 unit per 3–4 g of glucose). When available, the human or synthetic STH administration seems to be indicated during the first two postburn weeks, when the STH response to insulin induced hypoglycemia is minimal or just nil (stimulation of anabolism, improved fat mobilization, improved general resistance [10]). REN and ANGIO II levels, but especially the REN levels are probably important indicators of the general status of kidneys, of fluids and electrolytes (and catecholamine release?) in the burned. Their persisting high levels are definitely an unfavorable sign. New drugs and therapeutic procedures could be tested in the same patient with the use of plasma ACTH, REN and ANGIO II level estimation, as it was done with the neuroplegic M2 mixture.

Summary

After major burns, the increased mean fasting immunoreactive insulin (IRI) plasma levels persisted for 7 weeks. During glucose tolerance tests, a decreased glucose tolerance and increased insulin resistance (higher IRI response) were found. During the first 2 postburn weeks the STH response after insulin provoked hypoglycemia was practically blocked, it increased above normal in the later weeks. The fasting STH levels after burns were somewhat increased, especially in the second postburn month. High or even very high plasma renin (REN) and angiotensin II (ANGIO II) levels persisted even for more weeks in severely burned patients (the highest REN value found was 37 ng/ml/hr). The response of the renin-angiotensin system was increased during walking after major burns. Very high ACTH plasma levels were found in major burns, they persisted for a few postburn weeks and attained sometimes the levels found in the central form of the Cushing syndrome (e.g. 1 200 pg/ml). The increase of ACTH levels during a day was successfully blocked by the neuroplegic M2 mixture. In the patients studied the LH plasma levels were not decreased in the first postburn weeks.

The use of crystalline insulin is advocated after burns, the use of homologous STH is substantiated in the first postburn weeks. The REN, ANGIO II and ACTH levels could be used to test the efficiency of new drugs and therapeutic procedures after burns.

The study included 45 burned patients, with the mean burn index of 32.8 points.

References

1. ALLISON, S. P., HINTON, P. and CHAMBERLAIN, M. J. (1968): Intravenous glucose tolerance, insulin and free-fatty-acid levels in burned patients. Lancet 2 : 1113.
2. ARTZ, C. P. and MONCRIEF, J. A. (1969): The Treatment of Burns, 2nd Ed. Saunders Co, Philadelphia.
3. BOŽOVIĆ, L., CASTENFORTH, J., EKLUND, J., GRANBERG, P. O. and LILJEDAHL, S. O. (1967): Plasma-renin activity in burned patients. Lancet 1 : 574.
4. DOLEČEK, R., BUSE, M. and KUPERMINC, D. (1969): Insulin and growth hormone levels after burns. Čas. Lék. čes. 108 : 1520.
5. DOLEČEK, R., KALINA, J. et al. (1970): Léčení popálených (The Treatment of the Burned), Avicenum, Praha.
6. DOLEČEK, R., ZÁVADA, M., BEŠKA, F. and BURYŠKOVÁ, D. (1971): Immunoreactive insulin and growth hormone plasma levels after burns. Rozhl. Chir. 50: 577.
7. DOLEČEK, R., ZÁVADA, M., BEŠKA, F. and BURYŠKOVÁ, D. (1972): Plasma immunoreactive and growth hormone levels in burned subjects. Acta chir. plast. 14 : 179.
8. DOLEČEK, R., ZÁVADA, M., ADÁMKOVÁ, M. and LEIKEP, K. (1973): Plasma renin like activity (RLA) and angiotensin II levels after major burns. Acta chir. plast. 5 : 166.
9. DOLEČEK, R., ZÁVADA, M., ADÁMKOVÁ, M. and LEIKEP, K. (1973): Plasma ACTH, renin and angiotensin II levels after burns. Čas. Lék. čes. (in press).
10. SELYE, H. (1971): Hormones and Resistance. Springer, Berlin.

R. D., Urxova 2, 70 800 Ostrava 8,
Czechoslovakia

CONTEMPORARY CHANGES IN THE CLINICAL PRESENTATION OF THE BURN DISEASE

J. NOVAK

Clinic for Burn Diseases, Budapest, Hungary

In the course of the last decades, the overall character, clinical presentation, and complications of the burn disease have been undergoing many changes. Till the Second World War, cachexia was an almost inevitable complication of severe burn disease. Gram-positive microbial sepsis was a frequent phenomenon, to say nothing about circulatory insufficiency.

Penicillin, streptomycin, and finally broad-spectrum antibiotics, increasingly active surgical treatment, and mainly the discovery of the important role played by the water balance and energic metabolic processes in the inception and duration of the burn disease — all this brought about changes in the clinical presentation and course of the burn disease. At our clinic, we treated, in the course of recent years, 1700 burn victims, of whom 120 died. If Rittenbury's index were applied, the number of deaths would be 138. At autopsy of the 120 patients who had died we found gastric and duodenal ulcers in four, which corresponds to only 2 per mille of the total number of 1700 patients. Besides, in six autopsied patients we found mucosal erosion (4 per mille). In two patients, preexisting gastric ulcers became activated, but healed again later on. Similarly, thanks to modern methods of treatment, renal insufficiency has lost its former dangerousness.

In the course of the last decades, septicaemia and sepsis caused by gram-positive microbes have been displaced by invasive infections by gram-negative microbes. Since we had learned to recognize in time the characteristic features of this severe complication, the number of mycotic infections has been increasing.

At our clinic we have encountered this complications only rarely, no doubt because we administer antibiotics only occasionally, for short periods, and in strictly indicated cases only. Within the last two years, we diagnosed a mycotic infection in as few as six patients altogether. In five of them, the mycotic skin infection was a sequela of mycosis preexisting already before the burn accident.

Heart failure, one of well-known complications of burn disease, was rare (0.2 per mille) at our burn treatment centre thanks to an early mobilization, for which credit is due to active surgical treatment. In three cases we concluded that surgery had been delayed, and in consequence the patients were confined to bed for long periods. In a single case, an early mobilization of the patient had to be interrupted owing to imminent cardiac decompensation. We wish to comment that cardiac pharmacostimulation has not as yet found wide application in our country. The early mobilization of patients also explains the fewness of thromboembolic complications. Out of the total number of 1700 patients, lung embolism was the cause of death in 16 patients (1 per cent). In another 11 patients (0.6 per cent), thrombosis of lower limbs was found at the autopsy. Seven surviving patients with lower limb thrombosis healed completely; in six patients the postthrombotic syndrome persisted. In five of these patients, leg ulcers developed, and two of the patients had to be operated upon several years later.

One patient suffered myocardial infarction, because of which his rehabilitation was postponed for 1.5 months.

In connexion with prolonged venous drip infusions, in 13 patients there developed phlebitis at the entrance of the intravenous cannula; six of these patients had suffered burns by electric current. The relatively low incidence of complications of this type may be explained by our replacing the intravenous catheter even repeatedly, if necessary.

All these data show that in the total number of 1700 hospitalized patient with the burn disease, thromboembolic complications occurred in 2 per cent, and inclusive of the cases of phlebitis, in 3 per cent of the patients. In our opinion, these favourable results are ascribable to timely replacement of the destroyed skin (by preserved skin in the given case), as well as to early surgery and mobilization. We add that we administer anticoagulants only in established thrombosis of large veins.

Mental disturbances in burn victims have been increasing in number. We explain this phenomenon by an increase in the frequency of thermal injuries, which are accompanied, as a rule, by severe mental stress.

Unfortunately, anaemia has remained an inevitable complication of the burn disease. Clinical observations by Bernath proved that the suppression of erythropoiesis is due to a disturbance of iron metabolism, caused in turn by prolonged stress. So far, no causal method of treatment is available which would directly repair the disturbed metabolism of iron, and blood transfusions have to be resorted to.

Nowadays, the course of burn disease is incontestably more favourable than in the past. In our opinion, credit for this is due primarily to the continually spreading use of early (in the first days) and late surgery. We wish to point out, in particular, the positive role of tangential excision.

In our opinion, the prime factor capable to further improve an unfavourable clinical course of the burn disease would be a successful causal treatment of anaemia.

J. N., Stáhly u. 2/A,
1085 Budapest, Hungary

PRODUCTION OF THE ENDOGENOUS ERYTHROPOIETIN IN BURNED RATS AND ITS INFLUENCE BY ANAEMISATION AND TESTOSTERONE

J. VAŇÁSEK and J. MAZÁK

Second Department of Medicine Faculty of Medicine, Charles University, Hradec Králové, Czechoslovakia

In the course of the serious burns-disease a clinically significant anaemia develops. The pathogenesis is complicated and not well known and the therapy is only substitutional.

The aim of the work was to study the possible participation of changes of endogenous erythropoietin production in the development of anaemia and in a later stage of experiment to study the possibility to influence therapeutically the erythropoietin production.

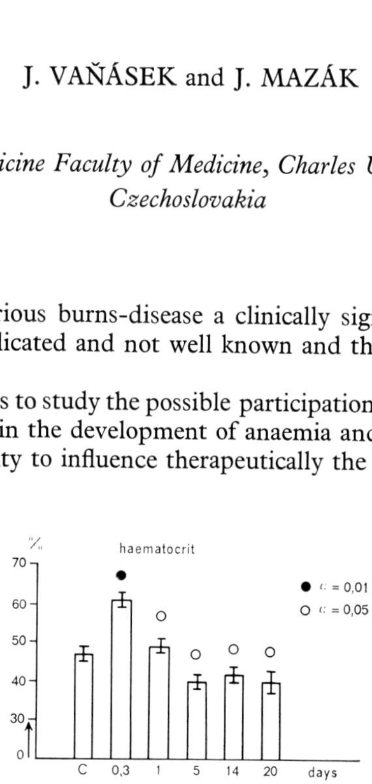

Fig. 1. Haematocrit in rats with 30 per cent body surface area burned.

Male white rats, to whom third degree burns of 35 per cent of the body surface were inflicted, were used. The haematocrit and haemoglobin level, the erythrocytes, reticulocytes and leukocytes counts, myelogram, the absolute cellularity of the bone marrow and the absolute cellularity of separate lines in the bone marrow were examined in the period 8 and 24 hours, 5, 14 and 20 days after the burn. Simultaneously, the level of the endogenous erythropoietin was determined by modification of the method of Nečas and Živný. During the experimental work 10 mg of streptomycin and 10.000 U of procaine penicillin were intramuscularly applied to rats with the aim to reduce the secondary infection and decrease its effect on haemopoiesis.

The experiment was carried out on the following series of rats:

- burned rats only;
- anaemized burned rats. Anaemisation was carried out by cardial puncture of 4 ml 24 hours before sacrificing;
- burned rats with intraperitoneal application of 1 mg free testosterone immediately after the burn and further with subcutaneous injection of 1 mg testosterone propionate applied every other day. In case of rats killed 8 and 24 hours after the burn, testosterone was applied already 72–96 hours before sacrificing the animals in order to influence haemopoiesis;
- burned rats anaemized immediately and treated by testosterone.

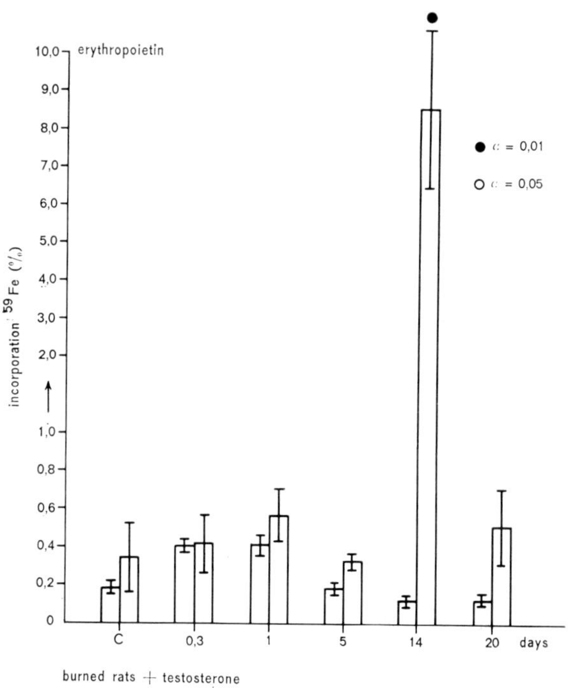

Fig. 2. Erythropoietin level in blood plasma of burned rats (^{59}Fe incorporation in erythrocytes of control polycythaemic mice—first column, and in mice given blood plasma of burned rats — second column).

In the experiment with burned rats only the chosen model of burn evoked haemoconcentration after 8 hours; it disappeared after 24 hours and was followed by anaemia lasting until the end of the experiment (the 20th day) (Fig. 1).

In spite of anaemia of burned rats, the level of the erythropoietin was low with the exception of values obtained on the 5th day after the burn when the level increased temporarily (Fig. 2). In the graph, in a couple of columns, the first shows always the intensity of ^{59}Fe incorporation in the control polycythemic mice. The second column shows the incorporation after the application of tested plasma of the burned rats.

Fig. 3 demonstrates that anaemisation only (without the burn) causes a highly significant increase of erythropoietin. If the rats are burned, the increase of the level of erythropoietin appears, but in this case the stimulation by anaemisation does not develop as markedly as in the control non-burned animals. This suggests that after the burn the organism has a lower ability to increase the level of erythropoietin after stimulation by anaemisation.

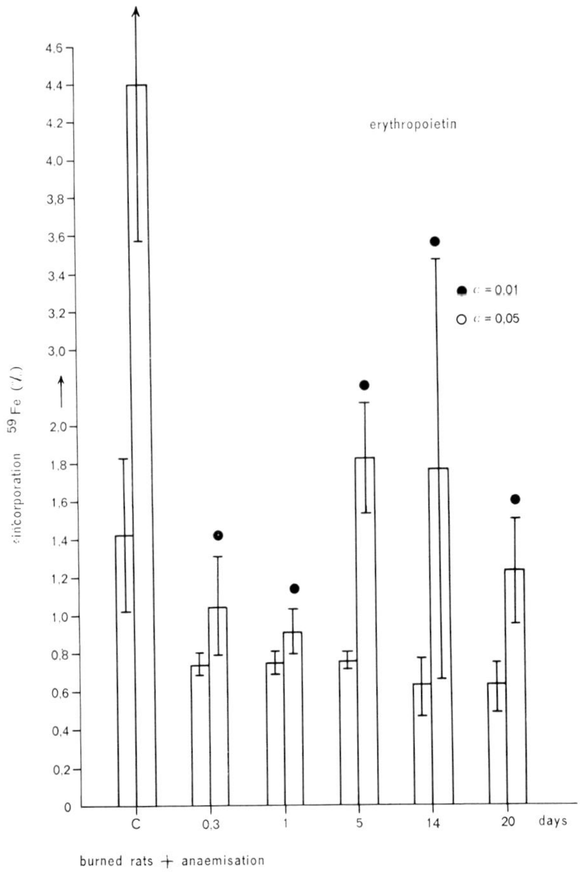

Fig. 3. Erythropoietin level in blood plasma of burned and anaemised rats.

In burned rats with testosterone application the level of erythropoietin is increased in the series during the later period of the experiment. But this increase is not too significant with the exception of the period of the 14th day (Fig. 4).

Fig. 5 demonstrates the important increase of the level of erythropoietin in all rats burned, anaemized and simultaneously treated by testosterone.

On the basis of the above-mentioned results, which are in correlation with the other investigated values, we believe that it may be concluded:

1. the influence of erythropoietin participates in the development of the postburn anaemia beside other known factors;

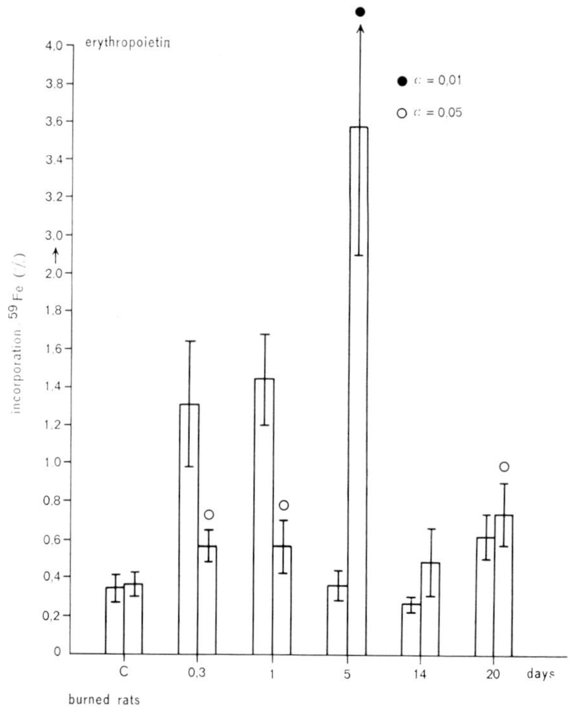

Fig. 4. Erythropoietin level in blood plasma of burned rats given testosterone.

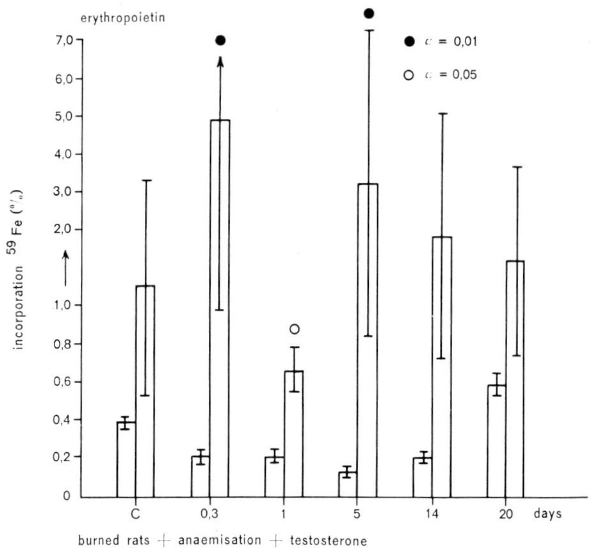

Fig. 5. Erythropoietin level in blood plasma of burned and anaemised rats given testosterone.

2. in the course of the burn the organism has a lower ability to react to stimuli of anaemisation by an increase in the erythropoietin level;

3. the application of testosterone alone during the burn disease causes only a low increase of erythropoietin production;

4. the combination of stimuli by anaemisation and testosterone causes a significant increase in erythropoietin production.

We suppose that the importance of erythropoietin for the development and course of the postburn anaemia should be further investigated as the therapeutical influence on the level of erythropoietin could in the future contribute to causal treatment of postburn anaemia.

J. V., 2nd Dept. of Medicine,
Pospíšilova tř.,
500 00 Hradec Králové, Czechoslovakia

ICTERUS IN BURN ILLNESS

J. CHLUMSKÝ, R. VRABEC, A. CHLUMSKÁ and B. MAREČEK

First Clinic of Internal Medicine, Burns Centre, and Institute of Pathological Anatomy, Faculty of Hygiene, Charles University, Prague, Central Customs Administration, Medical Department, Prague, Czechoslovakia

In the past, little attention was paid to icterus, which may appear at any stage of burn illness. Jaundice in burned patients was first described, as late as 1938, by Wilson, McGregor and Steward. For a long time it was believed that it had an infectious aetiology. A new classification was proposed in 1966 by Antonov. Our experience corresponds, by and large, with his conclusions.

As we have demonstrated in a previous study, secondary liver impairment develops relatively early after injury, but in most cases it becomes clinically apparent only at the beginning of the septic or toxemia stage. Its main signs are, as a rule, a slightly enlarged liver, a higher serum transaminase activity — not above the 200 mU/ml level — and a mild hyperbilirubinemia with values up to 5 mg per cent, found practically in 80 per cent of all burned patients. Histological findings usually correspond to dystrophic hepatic changes of various degrees.

Given these results, we were able to eliminate a viral aetiology of such liver damage and to consider this kind of icterus as an integral symptom of a secondary hepatic lesion due to the burn disease and its complications. This was further confirmed by a negative Au-antigen, regularly investigated in all patients.

For the same reasons there could exceptionally occur, as Antonov has already stressed, an acute flaring-up of a chronic hepatic disorder, which till then may have developed only latently.

The above mentioned findings are of considerable practical importance. Not so long ago, patients with this frequent jaundice were fairly often transferred to an infectious ward and thus removed from the care of plastic surgeons and their medical collaborators, specialised in the treatment of this type of injury. It need not be stressed that this was usually to the detriment of the patients.

On the other hand, we may get 3 to 4 months after injury, and even later, a late icterus with sufficiently typical clinical and laboratory symptoms of viral hepatitis, probably of a serum type. Since it attacks hepatic tissue recently damaged during the burn disease, such an infection may have a severe, protracted course and possibly even a lethal ending.

We have observed viral hepatitis in 7 cases, i.e. in 17.5 per cent of all patients under observation. Late clinical and biopsy check-ups revealed in 2 out of the 7 patients a transition from acute hepatic impairment to chronic hepatitis. And, finally, fulminant viral hepatitis in a 50 year old obese diabetic woman patient, in a late convalescence stage of burns illness, ended in a hepatic coma, which resisted all treatment.

Summary

Mild jaundice in 80 per cent of the observed cases may indicate hepatic damage, which occurs almost regularly already during the first week in every more severe and extensive burn disease. This early icterus, a symptom of hepatic damage caused directly by the burn injury or by other noxious influences, must not be mistaken for a late icterus which does not, as a rule, appear until the 3rd or 4th month after injury, or even later, and which is mostly caused by viral hepatitis, probably of a serum type. The serious complications of this infection are stressed.

References

1. Antonov, V. B. (1966): Klinika i patogenez zheltukh u ozhzhenykh. Voenuomed. Zh. 10 : 47.
2. Chlumský, J., Vrabec, R., Mareček, B. and Chlumská, A.: Klinický obraz jaterního poškození u popáleninové nemoci. Acta chir. plast. (in print).
3. Colson, P., Gangolphe, M., Leclerq, P. et Honot, R. (1955): Hépatite grave chez un grand brulé — la méthode de Mowkur-Jackson. Lyon chir. 55 : 754.
4. Wartman, W. B. (1962): Mechanism of death in severe burn injury: The need for planned autopsies. In: Research in Burns. Amer. Inst. Biol. Sci,. Washington and Blackwell Scient. Publ., Oxford, 9 : 6.

J. C., Ist Internal Clinic,
Šrobárova 50,
100 34 Praha 10, Czechoslovakia

CLINICAL PICTURE OF LIVER DAMAGE IN BURN ILLNESS

J. CHLUMSKÝ, R. VRABEC, A. CHLUMSKÁ and B. MAREČEK

First Clinic of Internal Medicine, Burns Centre, Plastic Surgery, Institute of Pathological Anatomy, Faculty of Hygiene, Charles University, Prague, Central Customs Administration, Medical Department, Prague, Czechoslovakia

Already at the end of the last century, Schjerning (1884) and Bardeen (1898) had pointed out the presence of liver changes in thermal skin damage. However, only a new approach to the problem of burns, rightly considered today as a general disease affecting all vital functions, the solution of some basic questions of treatment, as well as advances in hepatological diagnostics gave us the possibility to study in full the role of the liver in burn illness.

TABLE 1

Patients' age and sex

Age	11–20	21–30	31–40	41–50	51–60	61–70	71–80	81–90	Total
Men	7	13	6	1	2	0	2	1	32
Women	1	1	1	3	1	1	0	0	8
Total	8	14	7	4	3	1	2	1	40

TABLE 2

Causes of death in 12 patients

Causes of Death	No.
Sepsis or toxaemia	5
Heart-failure	5
Shock	1
Liver-failure	1

Since January 1971, we have carried out clinical and laboratory investigations of 40 patients treated for more severe forms of thermal skin damage in the intensive care unit of our faculty Burns Centre. In 30 patients hepatic tissue samples obtained by a puncture technique according to Menghini were also examined. Table 1 gives our patients' age and sex. The mean age of the men was 32.7 years and of the women 41.1 years. The extent of burns, assessed mainly as burns of the 2nd and 3rd and only rarely of the 4th degree, was 46.5 per cent in the men and 54.4 per cent in the women of their body surface. From the above mentioned number of patients 12 persons died. The extent of their burns was approximately 10 per cent higher than in the survivors. Causes of deaths are given in Table 2, the most frequent being sepsis or heart-failure; on the other hand shock and other complications were relatively rare.

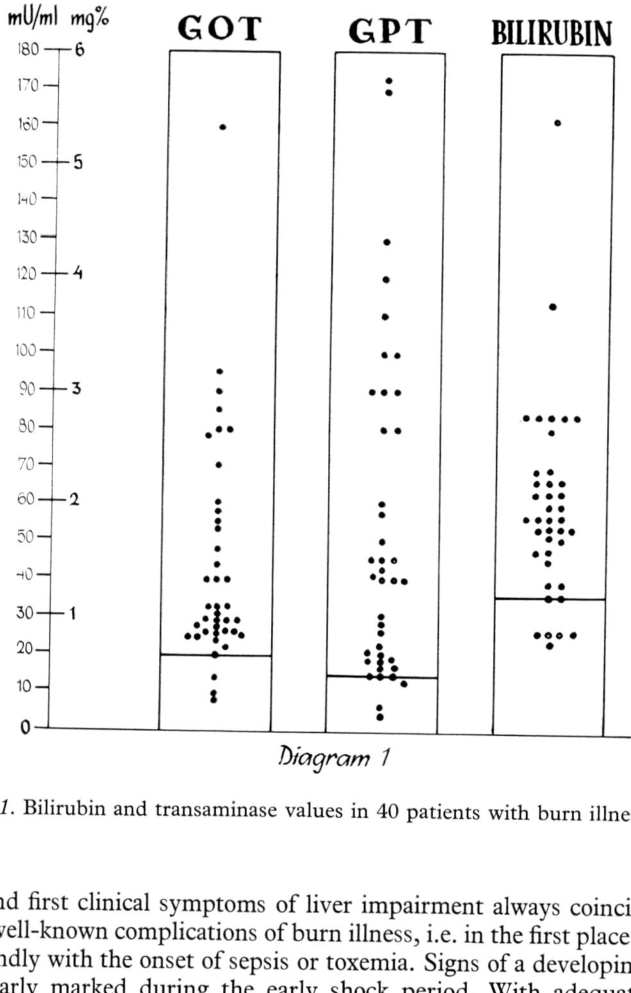

Fig. 1. Bilirubin and transaminase values in 40 patients with burn illness.

The onset and first clinical symptoms of liver impairment always coincided with the appearance of well-known complications of burn illness, i.e. in the first place with signs of shock and secondly with the onset of sepsis or toxemia. Signs of a developing liver lesion were never clearly marked during the early shock period. With adequate anti-shock treatment they need not appear at all. Thus higher serum transaminases were observed only twice.

The participation of the liver in the clinical picture of burn illness becomes, as a rule, obvious only from the 3rd to 7th day onwards, when the septic or toxemia stage begins. Of gastro-intestinal, often polymorphous, symptoms such as anorexia, nausea, more seldom vomiting or diarrhea, which may be present, perhaps only pressure in the right subcostal region can be taken for the first sign of developing hepatopathy. During that time we usually found a slightly enlarged liver — one to two fingers above the costal arch. We have frenquently observed a rise in the serum transminases GOT and GPT — within the range 25–100 mU/ml, rarely up to 170 mU/ml. Relatively soon after injury we obser-

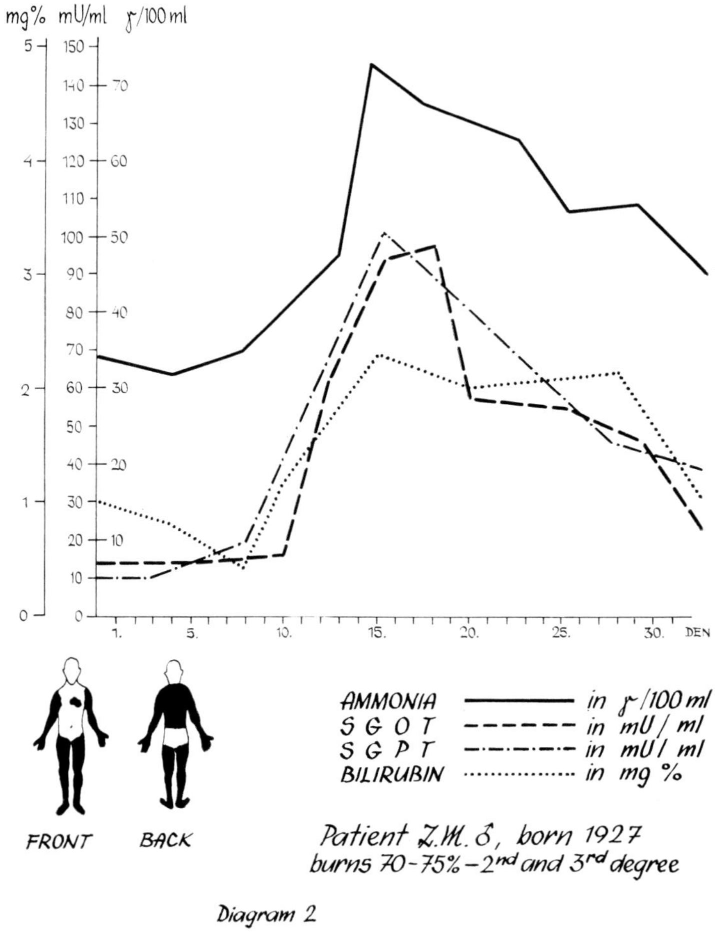

Fig. 2. Some laboratory values during the toxemia stage of burn illness.

ved higher bilirubin levels in the serum — in 80 per cent of all cases under observation. Hyperbilirubinemia was, as a rule, only slight — never above 5 mg per cent (Fig. 1).

In 8 patients we did a long-term follow-up of blood ammonia levels. In all there appeared — although somewhat later as compared with all other tests — a slight hyperammonemia either at the height of toxemia or with the first signs of its receding; it decreased, however, later with the decreasing serum transaminase activity and bilirubinemia Fig. 2.

Discussion

Our experience to date has once more confirmed that hepatic damage is always involved in the clinical picture of all more severe and extensive burn illnesses. But given the localisation of skin lesions and often also the lack of satisfactory cooperation of the patient, we can rely neither on subjective complaints nor on physical signs of an enlarged liver. It is always necessary to carry out some reliable laboratory tests.

Although secondary liver impairment appears early after injury, it is fairly subdued, both clinically and morphologically, during the shock period. Hepatic changes become more pronounced with the onset of sepsis or toxemia. However, they never attain the same degree as in viral hepatitis, which presents an entirely different clinical picture and appears at a different period.

The aetiology of secondary hepatic damage is undoubtedly multifactorial. During the period of shock, whose negative influence can be reduced to a minimum by modern antishock treatment, we may encounter hepatic tissue ischemia, due to impaired circulation in the splanchnic and intrahepatic regions. To this must be added the loss of fluids and proteins, as well as a disturbed electrolytic and acidobasic balance usually leading to acidosis. Simultaneously, there is a drop in energy metabolism. Later, due to the resorption of tissue and toxin disintegration products, an increased load is put on the disintoxication functions of the liver and on the hepatic RES. Microbial gram-negative infection is largely responsible for the prolonged existence and, possibly, for the increase of metabolic disturbances and for the failure of homoestatic and defence mechanisms. The list of potential harmful factors would be incomplete, were we to omit the possible influence of anesthesia, the load represented by repeated surgical interventions and sometimes perhaps even the unfavourable hepatotrophic effect of some highly effective antibiotics, essential for an efficient fight against sepsis, a regular companion of all extensive skin lesions.

All this enables us to draw conclusions for a complex therapy, which should also include the stimulation of liver functions, as a rule impaired in burn illness.

Summary

In 40 patients with severe forms of burn illness we have studied the clinical picture of secondary liver damage, which only rarely appears during the shock period, but almost always during the septic or toxemia stage. We also mention the aetiopathogenesis of secondary liver impairment. A complex therapy of burn illness must include a stimulation of hepatic functions.

References

1. Chlumský, J., Vrabec, R., Mareček, B. and Chlumská, A.: Klinický obraz jaterního poškození u popáleninové nemoci (Clinical Picture of Liver Damage in Burn Illness). Acta Chir. plast. (in print).
2. Creyssel, J., Deleuze, R., Gaté, A. and Savignac, A. (1964): Incidences des brûlures sur les fonctions hépatiques. Lyon chir. 60 : 575.
3. Sternberg, T. and Hogeman, K. E. (1962): Experimental and clinical investigations on liver function in burns. In: Research in Burns. Amer. Inst. Biol. Sci., Washington, and Blackwell Scientific Publications, Oxford, 9 : 171.
4. Zimmermann, W. E., Bennert, C., Knote, G., and Mittermayer, C. (1969): Funktionelle und biochemische Veränderungen des retikuloendothelialen Systems der Leber beim Verbrennungsschock und deren mögliche Auswirkung auf die Infektion. In: Verbrennungskrankheit. F. K. Schattauer Verlag, Stuttgart-New York, 35.

J. C., Ist Internal Clinic,
Šrobárova 50,
100 34 Praha 10, Czechoslovakia

MORPHOLOGICAL FINDINGS IN HEPATIC TISSUE OF BURNED PATIENTS

A. CHLUMSKÁ, J. DOBIÁŠ and J. CHLUMSKÝ

Institute of Pathological Anatomy and 1st Clinic of Internal Medicine, Faculty of Hygiene, Charles University, Prague, Czechoslovakia

We have studied hepatic tissue changes in 45 burned patients, aged 10 to 88 years. Puncture samples were taken 1 day to 2.5 years after injury, 18 samples up to 3 hours after death. The burns ranged from 9 to 80 per cent of the total body surface area, with an average of 45 per cent, and were predominantly of the 2nd and 3rd degree. In 10 patients microscopic examinations of hepatic tissue were repeated after 14 to 315 days.

For these examinations current histological techniques were used.

During the first week after the burn injury, we have examined 6 patients — in hepatic tissue with a preserved structure we found irregular nuclei in hepatocytes with large nucleoli and vacuolised nuclei. Hepatic cells very often had voluminous, light-coloured, balloonlike plasma, poor in glycogen, and a regularly dispersed unicellular or focal steatosis in the form of small droplets or large globules, mainly localised on the acini periphery. Kupffer's cells were either focally or diffusely activated, sometimes with plasma vacuolisation. Regressive changes in Kupffer's cells were observed only exceptionally.

In 2 patients with a slight fibrosis of portobiliary spaces and with non-healing septal fibroses, hepatic cells decayed either individually or in small groups.

From the second week after injury onwards, we noticed in the hepatic tissue, besides focal steatosis, resorbtive nodes around the decaying hepatocytes, an activation of Kupffer's cells and sometimes round-cell infiltrations of portobiliary spaces. These changes prevailed for long periods: in 1 case they were still present 2.5 years after injury.

In cases with more extensive burns, complicated by a prolonged septic state, we found pronounced dystrophic hepatic tissue changes with the presence of large hepatocytes, diffuse steatosis and focal hepatic cell necrosis, usually localised contra-acinosely.

After the 11th day, we have observed a post-transfusion hemosiderosis of Kupffer's cells and, to some extent, even of hepatic cells on the acini periphery.

In seven patients, convalescence was complicated 3 to 3.5 months after burning by infectious hepatitis, probably of a serum type. Biopsy, done 6 weeks to 6 months after the appearance of first hepatitis signs, revealed in 4 cases a portobiliary and mildly septal fibrosis and in 3 cases an active hepatitis.

In assessing our findings, we can say that hepatic tissue damage during the early post-burn period, when shock changes prevail, corresponds to an increased metabolic hepatocyte activity, appearing morphologically as enlarged nucleoli often localised along the edges of different sized, partly vacuolised nuclei and as dystrophic changes in the form of swollen hepatic cell plasma poor in glycogen. Further, we have regularly encountered unicellular to focal steatosis, localised mainly on the acini periphery. Only in 2 elderly patients with fibrosis and a relatively small cornered deformation of portobiliary spaces, which bespeaks older hepatic tissue damage, did we find during that period a dispersed decay of individual hepatocytes. Contrary to some data in literature, hepatic tissue changes during the first post-burn week were relatively small, thus confirming an effective anti-shock therapy.

From the second week onwards, we found more pronounced dystrophic hepatic cell changes, mostly of a focal nature, and in 4 patients even diffuse steatosis. Further, we regularly encountered dispersed to focal hepatocyte decay. The above mentioned changes can be seen a long time after thermal injury, although they partly lose their intensity during burn illness convalescence.

Hepatic tissue damage depended on the extent and degree of burns, but was present even in smaller burns. It depended also on the patients' age and the post-burn period, when further negative influences came into play, especially sepsis or toxemia, repeated anesthesia and surgical interventions.

Infectious hepatitis — probably of a serum type — diagnosed in 7 patients 3 to 3.5 months after injury, always had a serious clinical course. In no case did we observe healing ad integrum and in 3 cases we found a transition into a subacute or chronic stage.

Summary

Morphological changes in puncture samples of hepatic tissue from 45 burned patients were, during the first week after injury, in the nature of dystrophic changes, mainly in the form of steatosis. At a later stage, besides more pronounced dystrophic changes, decay of hepatic cells was also confirmed.

References

1. Benaim, F., Fattin, M. and Rappaport, M. (1962): Puncture Biopsy of the Liver in Critical Burns. In: Research in Burns. Amer. Inst. Biol. Sci., Washington, and Blackwell Scientific Publications, Oxford, 9 : 185.
2. Bednář, B., Schön, E. and Soušek, O. (1965): Akutní virová hepatitida a její následky. (Acute viral hepatitis and its consequences). Čs. Patol. 1 : 3.
3. Ionescu, A., Chiotan, N. and Paulian, V. (1969): Intravital and post-mortem study of liver structure changes in the burned. Panminerva med. 11 : 47.

A. C., Inst. of Pathological Anatomy,
Šrobárova 50,
100 34 Praha 10, Czechoslovakia

TREATMENT OF RESPIRATORY INSUFFICIENCY IN BURNED PATIENTS

G. GRIGOROV, Y. EMANUILOV, B. TORLAKOVA and A. KRASTEV

Emergency Medical Institute N. I. Pirogov, Sofia, Bulgaria

The pulmonary complications in patients with extensive burns increased in the last few years, leading to a high mortality rate (1, 2, 3, 5).

Over the past 6 years we observed 50 patients with respiratory insufficiency at the age ranging from 10 months to 73 years and burned surface from 17 to 80 per cent. Only 6 of them had a direct damage of the respiratory tract due to the thermic agent. The sequelae of the haemodynamic disorders in the shock phase, the overadministration of fluids and the sepsis caused pulmonary complications in the other patients. They develop insidiously over a period of hours or days and are clinically obvious most frequently between the 3rd and 8th day after the burn. The progressive respiratory insufficiency passes through 4 phases:

1. latent,
2. prodromal,
3. marked,
4. severe respiratory and cardio-vascular decompensation.

The marked respiratory insufficiency is overcome with difficulty and the pulmonary changes are rarely reversible (congested, collapsed alveoli, loss of surfactant, and exudation of fluid, albumin and some destructive enzymes). All our patients in this phase died without having been influenced by the therapy applied. Only early preventive treatment (in the latent and prodromal phases) is able to stop the progressive character of the complication.

The following therapy has been applied:

1. Restriction of fluid therapy, using mainly colloid solutions (albumin — 5 and 20 per cent, plasma).

TABLE 1

Latent phase

1. Without clinical symptoms
2. Chest X-ray: congested pulmonary vasculature
3. Moderate hypoxamia — PaO_2 TO 75 mm.Hg
4. Moderate hypocarbia — $PaCO_2$ to 30 mm.Hg

TABLE 2

Prodromal phase

1. Restlessness
2. Tachypnoe — TO 30–35/min.
3. Chest X-ray: initial interstitial pulmonary oedema
4. Progressive hypoxaemia — PaO_2 below 75 mm.Hg
5. Progressive hypocarbia — $PaCO_2$ below 30 mm.Hg

TABLE 3

Effect of the Diuretic Therapy

Group	Issue	Died	Survived	Total
Without administration of diuretics	Number of patients	20	3	23
	per cent	87	13	
With administration of diuretics	Number of patients	12	15	27
	per cent	44.5	55.5	

TABLE 4

Indications for intubation

1. Dyspnoe
2. Tachypnoe — above 40/min.
3. Chest X-ray: progressive pulmonary oedema
4. PaO_2 – below 70 mm.Hg after 15 minutes breathing of 100 per cent O_2
5. $PaCO_2$ — above 60 mm.Hg
6. Increase in the dead space: Tidal volume ratio/V_D/V_T/above 0.6

TABLE 5

Interval between the onset of the marked respiratory insufficiency and the beginning of ventilation		1 day	2 days	3 days
Number of patients	Survived	5	3	0
		41.7 per cent	25 per cent	0 per cent
	Died	7	9	14
		58.3 per cent	75 per cent	100 per cent

2. Administration of diuretics – Furzemid, Polythiazid.
3. Oxygenotherapy.

During the latent phase oxygen is utilized only in progressive drop of PaO_2 about or below 70 mmHg, and in the prodromal phase – continuously maintaining PaO_2 between

80 and 100 mmHg. In adult patients the oxygen is given by means of a nasal catheter (a flow of 6 to 8 liters per minute) or by means of a mask (a flow of 8 to 10 liters per minute) and in children by means of an oxygen tent. Elevated oxygen tension for a prolonged period (over 48 hours) is avoided. If used continuously, its concentration must not exceed 40 per cent.

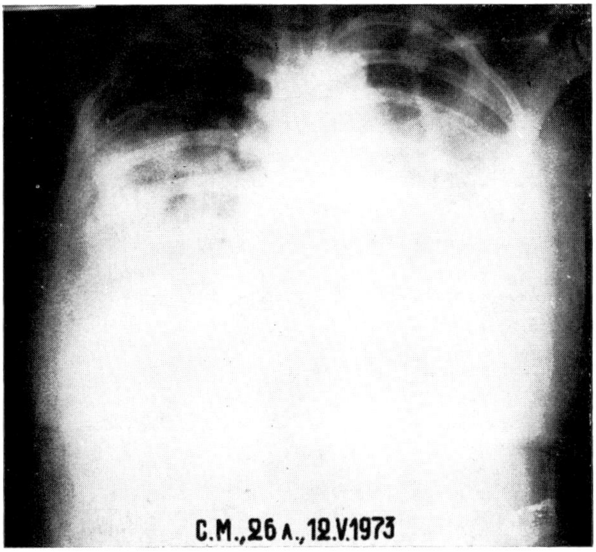

Fig. 1. 26-year-old female, 9 days after burn. Clinically obvious respiratory failure. Assisted ventilation required. Chest X-ray revealed areas of consolidation at the lung basis and in the left and right mid-zone.

In patients with extensive burns, the repeated arterial blood gas analysis is often difficult or impossible. In such cases the arterialized capillary sampling technique (method of Siggaard-Andersen and Engel with the Astrup micrometer) is routinely used.

4. Mechanical ventilation.
5. Humidification.

Bubble-type humidifiers are used when the patient is receiving oxygen through a catheter or mask (in cases where physiologic humidification mechanisms are utilized). For adequate humidification of patients with tracheostomies or endotracheal tubes we use nebulizers.

6. Frequent endotracheal suction.
7. Inhalation of mucolytics (mucosolvin), bronchodilators (aminophyllin, papaverin, isoprenaline) at an interval of 4 hours (for 30–60 minutes).
8. Chest physical therapy.

The diuretic therapy is essential in the early treatment of respiratory failure in our patients.

In the latent phase (Table 1) the drug of choice is Renese (polythiazide) at a dosage of 0.5–4 mg daily because of its prolonged diuretic and moderate saluretic effect. The patients with gastrointestinal paresis are given parenterally Furanthril (Furzemid). In the prodromal phase (Table 2) the dosage of the furzemid administered is increased to 480 mg daily.

In a group of 23 patients treated before the introduction of diuretic therapy, the morta-

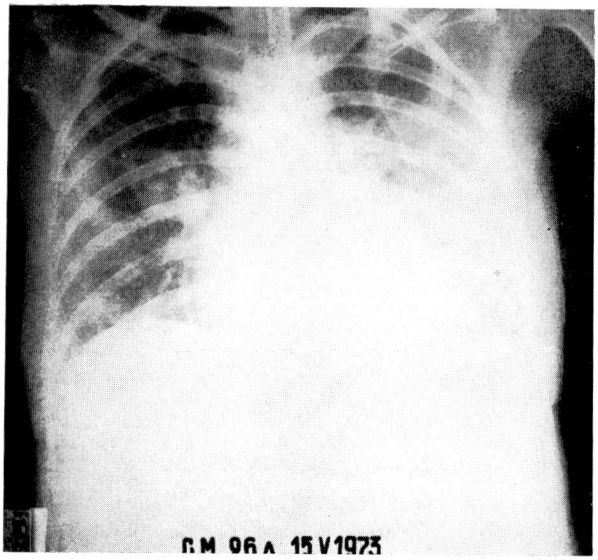

Fig. 2. Two days after beginning of the assisted ventilation. The improvement is insignificant.

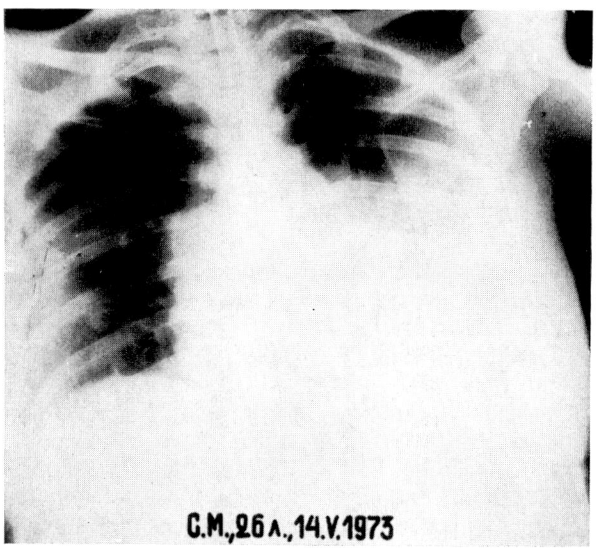

Fig. 3. On the next day after administration of 400 mg FURZEMID the area of consolidation in the lungs clears up rapidly.

lity rate was 87 per cent, and thereafter the mortality rate was decreased to 44.5 per cent in 27 patients. (Table 3).

When the respiratory failure is progressing and the parameters observed deteriorate (Table 4), we resort to mechanical ventilation with pressure limited respirators (Bird, Dräger-Assistor). All delay considerably increases the mortality rate (Table 5).

The best effect is obtained in combining the ventilation with diuretics (Fig. 1, 2, 3). Ventilation is used after previous intubation, most frequently nasotracheally under light anaesthesia. Patients with severe pulmonary failure are intubated without administration of depolarizing relaxants because of the danger of cardiac arrest. In order to obtain a sedative effect fractioned thalamonal is used, and in children sometimes ketalar. Muscle relaxants are administered to facilitate adequate ventilation in patients with rapid respiration or to achieve synchronization with the respirator.

In most of the patients, positive pressure breathing was applied. The ventilation is begun with a higher pressure ($+30$ to $+40/H_2O$) and after improvement of the blood gases the pressure is decreased. Every 10–15 minutes the lungs are inflated by means of a higher pressure (additionally $+10$ cm H_2O). In rapidly progressing respiratory failure continuous positive pressure breathing is used.

In the course of 10 days we ventilated patients without having any difficulty with the nasotracheal tube. In some cases who are treated with prolonged ventilation a tendency toward a positive water balance is observed after the 4th–5th day (syndrome described by Pontoppidan (4).

The weaning of the patient from artificial to spontaneous respiration must be gradual, in conformity with the breathing and the blood gases changes.

Tracheostomy is indicated in respiratory tract damage caused by a thermal agent (6 of our patients), prolonged intubation over 10 days and difficulty in the management of secretion. It must be always preceded by intubation.

References

1. Foley, F. D. (1969): The burn autopsy: fatal complications of burns. Amer. J. clin. Path. 52 : 1.
2. Jackson, T. M. and Lee, W. H. (1963): Major thermal burns: a mortality appraisal and review. Arch. Surg. 87 : 937.
3. Phillips, A. W. and Cope, O. (1962): Burn therapy. II. The revelation of respiratory tract damage as a principal killer of the burned patient. Ann. Surg. 155 : 1.
4. Pontoppidan, H. (1968): Treatment of respiratory failure in non-thoracic trauma. J. Trauma 8 : 938.
5. Silverstein, P., Dressler (1970): Effect of current therapy on burn mortality. Ann. Surg. 171 : 124.

G. G., Emergency Medical Inst.
„Pirogov“,
Sofia, Bulgaria

THE INFLUENCE OF BURNS ON JAW AND DENTURE DEVELOPMENT

J. KUFNER

Department of Maxillofacial Surgery of the Central Military Hospital, Prague, and Stomatological Department of the Faculty Hospital, Prague 10, Czechoslovakia

Face burns at juvenile age may affect the development of the jaws and denture.

This unfavourable influence is especially serious if burns affect the lips, the proximity of the mouth, the perimandibular, submandibular and upper neck regions.

The worst effect is exerted by burns at infantile age; as the child grows up the effect is smaller, and at adult age burns may not affect the denture and bite at all.

The development of the jaws and denture is the result of intraoral and extraoral formative forces. A disorder in the symmetry of these forces affects the further development of the jaws and denture. The pressure or traction of soft tissue scars exert an unfavourable influence on the further development of the part of jaw and denture pressed or drawn by the burn scars. Deeper burn scars, affecting even the muscles or the periosteum of the jaw, may directly impair the growth ability of the part involved. These negative influences result in asymmetric development of the denture and, often, even in a disorder in the intermaxillary relations.

Lower lip burns slow down the development of the lower dental arch and are responsible for the formation of pseudoprognathic bite.

Upper lip burns press upon the upper dental arch and the result is the formation of a reverse bite or even pseudoprogenia.

Scars in the perimandibular, submandibular and upper neck areas are responsible for asymmetric occlusion or even cross bite.

The traction of scars in the area of the chin may produce an open bite.

Scars in many other areas often lead to the combination of the described defects of bite and jaws at different degrees.

The purpose of this paper is to draw the attention of surgeons in burn departments to these facts, and to recommend that all children and teenagers affected by face burns should be sent to special dental (preferably orthodontic) departments in order to be subject to dispensary examination or, if necessary, to longer treatment.

Orthodontic treatment, in some cases supported by a surgical operation such as the removal of scars responsible for the worst pressure or traction, may prevent bite defects. The basic prerequisite is that orthodontic treatment should be started in time and carried out systematically.

Where the jaw and denture are already deformed, a stomatosurgical or sometimes also orthodontic intervention, followed by prosthetic treatment, may give favourable results.

Conclusion

Any face burn at infantile and juvenile age requires stomatological examination or even traetment. Surgeons at burn departments should bear this fact in mind.

J. K., Šrobárova 50,
101 00 Praha 10, Czechoslovakia

PSYCHOPATHOLOGIC PHENOMENA AND THEIR TREATMENT IN BURNS

P. PAVLOVSKÝ and P. POKORNÁ

Department of Psychiatry, Charles University, Prague, Czechoslovakia

Our paper is based on the results of the psychiatric examination and follow-up study of 323 in-patients of the Ward for burns of the Clinic for Plastic Surgery (Faculty Hospital in Prague 10) within the years 1967–1973. The average age of adult patients is 39 years, the set includes also 25 children.

In the course of burns we could encounter symptoms of neurotic and psychotic character.

During the first stage of burn disease patients complain about thirst, pain and disturbed sleep. In objective finding there is often some agitation and dominant thoughts about duties left unfulfilled. The mood is often slightly depressive with traits of anxiety. Consciousness is disturbed in severe burns only in the sense of gradual impairment from somnolence to sopor and coma, followed by death.

In the second stage various psychopathological phenomena can be seen. Depressive and anxiety states occur frequently, in several cases hypomanic syndrome appeared too. The basic symptom of psychotic states is disturbed consciousness. We speak about symptomatic psychoses the character of which is amentia or delirium syndromes. They appear mostly suddenly in evening hours of the second or third days after the injury. The patient is disorientated, anxious, and his perception is blurred. Highly agitated delirium states were seen in several alcoholic patients.

In the third stage we have met only neurotic symptoms as emotional lability, irritability, impatience, egocentrism, demanding, tiredness and insomnia.

In the fourth stage these symptoms did not mean a problem from the psychiatric point of view. An exception is represented by the patients who suffered severe burns with persistent consequences as cosmetic defects and impaired mobility. In some of these patients certain changes in their character appeared in the sense of increased introversion.

As we have already shown in our previous papers intensity of psychopathologic phenomena depends on severity of the injury, patient's age, his premorbid personality, appearance of mental disorders in his personal history and on his condition at the moment of the burn.

In many cases psychopathologic disturbances represented serious complications asking for special treatment.

As for psychotherapeutic methods the psychotherapeutic approach relieves fears of a new environment and surgical treatment, and to give an optimistic outlook is also neccessary. Hypnosis was used too and we find this method helpful in the cases of deep anxiety and fears of painful redressings.

In persistent serious defects we used systematic psychotherapy to rebuild the hierarchy of values to convince the patients about the neccessity and usefulness of their further existence diminishing their inferiority complex.

Early indemnity of work injuries is considered by us as an important preventive measure against long-lasting neurotic symptoms in certain cases.

Using drugs we concentrated especially at diazepam and chlorprothixen.

Diazepam (used preparations Seduxen and Faustan) was administered to 50 patients suffering from serious neurotic symptoms as complaints about hardly bearable pains, insomnia, obsessive worries, emotional disturbances and lack of collaboration with the nursing staff. In average diazepam was administered for three weeks in daily doses of 15 mg (5–40 mg). Improvement was often seen after two days of administration, especially in sleep disturbances (improvement in 76 per cent of cases): complaints about pains and worries became less excessive. Injections of Faustan were successful in delirious states of chronic alcoholics in daily doses of 40 mg.

Chlorprothixen was mainly used in anxiety-depressive states, in hard tension and insomnia and was given to 25 patients in average daily dosage of 30–60 mg for 5 weeks. Disturbed sleep was improved in 91 per cent, anxiety and depression in 62 per cent (while Seduxen was effective indication in 49 per cent).

In severe psychotic agitation we used chlorpromazin (preparation Plegomazin) intramuscularly in single dosis of 50–100 mg. In all 35 patients the agitation settled down. Thioridazin appeared less effective and doses of 75 mg in agitated elderly patients were too small.

As regards antidepressants we used Amitriptylin and Prothiaden in several cases of severe depressive reactions in daily dosage of 75 mg which brought improvement, mainly thanks to sedative effect of these drugs. Imipramin (Melipramin) was given in 8 cases of depression. Because of its rather late onset it appeared less helpful. In two cases of apathy-abulia syndrome some improvement was seen after daily doses of 75 mg. Dexfenmetrazin as a psychomimetic drug was also used in this indication but rather negative effects of insomnia, loss of appetite and irritability were seen.

In conclusion of our observation we can recommend drugs with psychopharmacological effects even in this medical field, as removing or diminishing of psychopathologic disturbances can speed up the healing process. The side effects of the drugs were mild and they did not bring about their premature discontinuation.

In our opinion psychiatric complications of burns ask for special treatment and the psychiatrist should be a member of specialists dealing with this disease.

P. P., Dept. of Psychiatry,
Ke Karlovu 11,
121 09 Praha 2, Czechoslovakia

AUTHORS' INDEX

* Numbers in bold types refer to the first page of the author's communication

SUBJECT INDEX